Periodontology - Fundamentals and Clinical Features

Edited by Petra Surlin

Published in London, United Kingdom

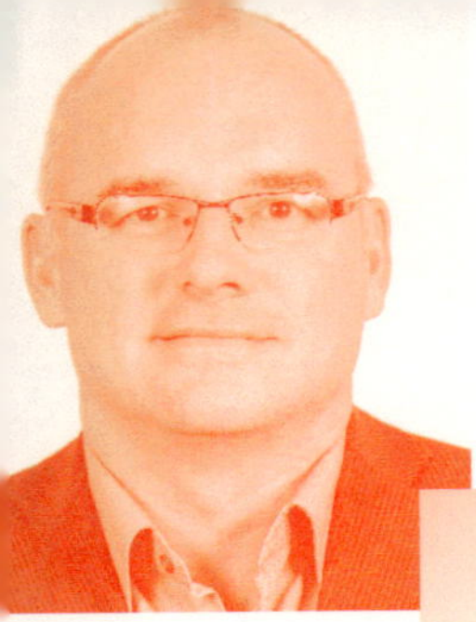
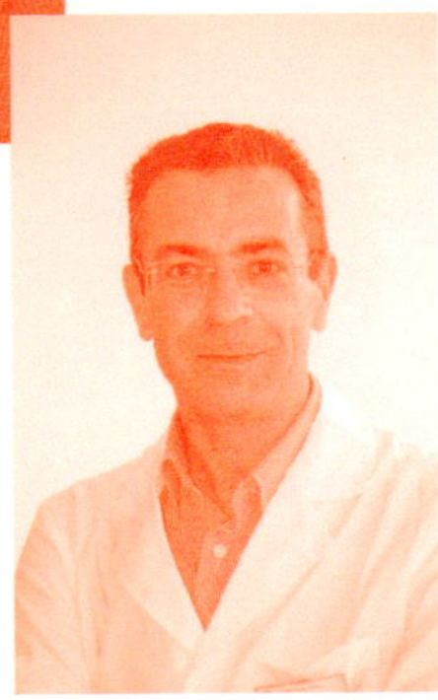
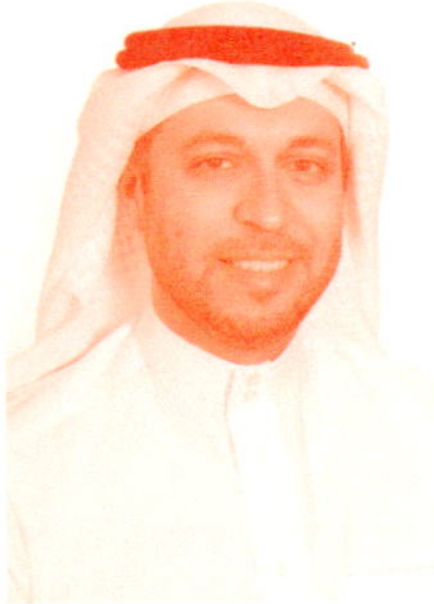
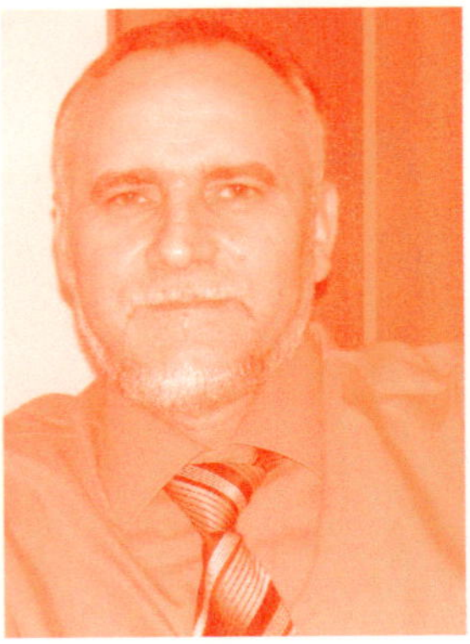
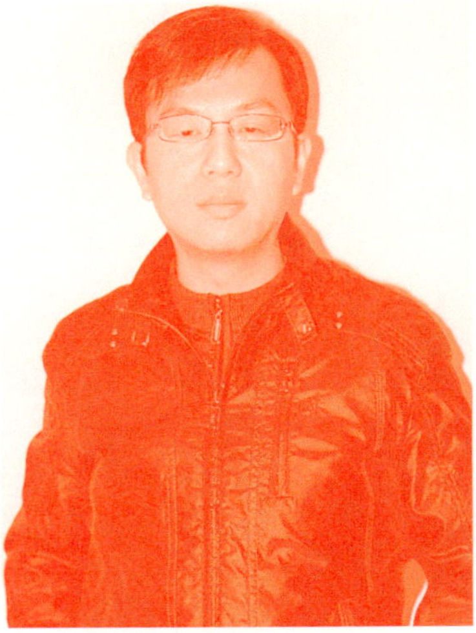
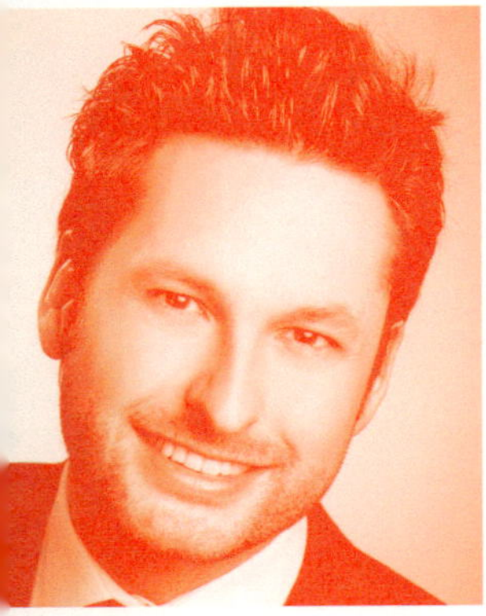
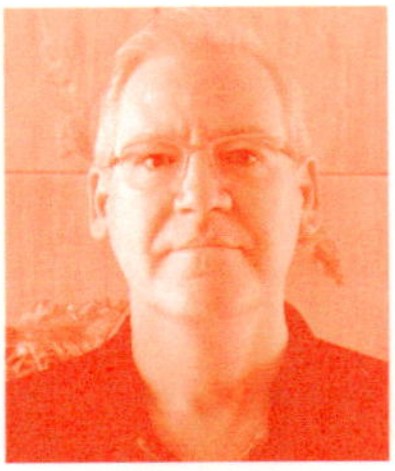

IntechOpen

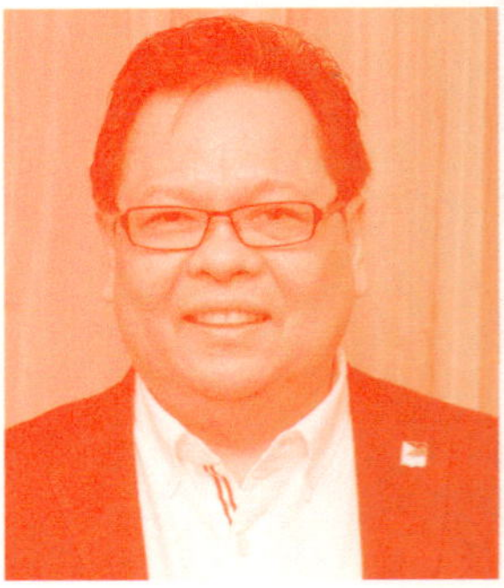
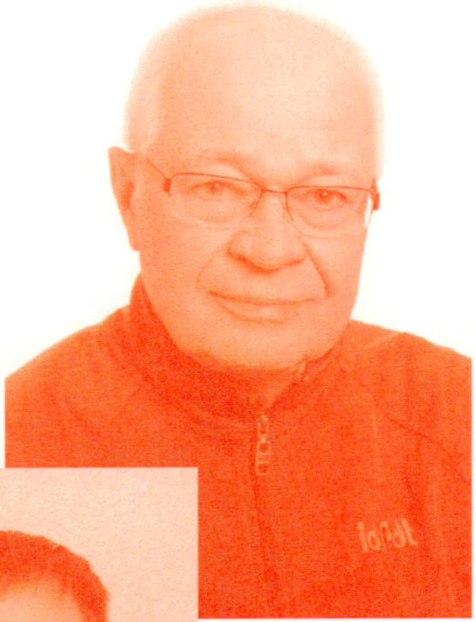
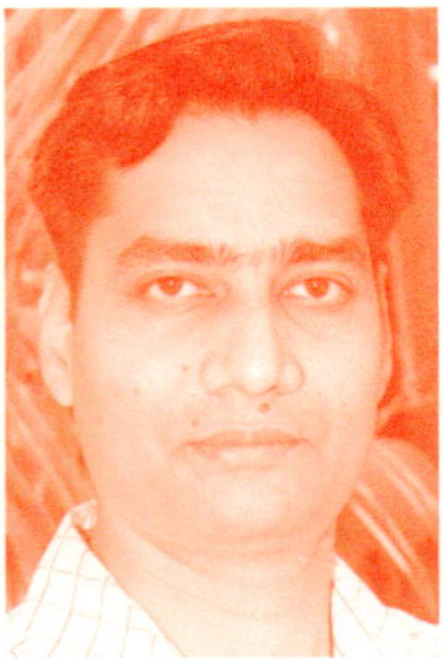
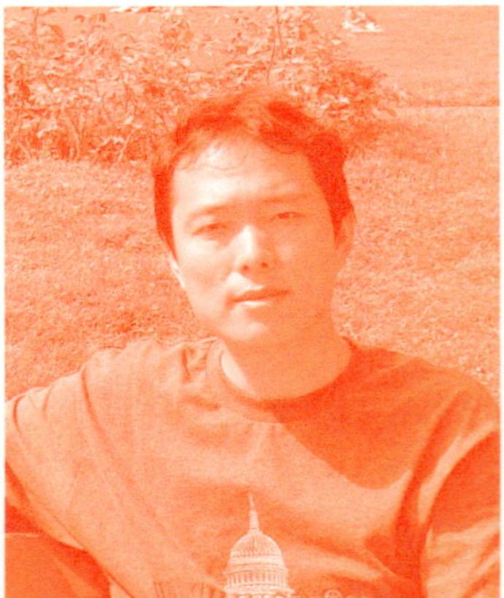
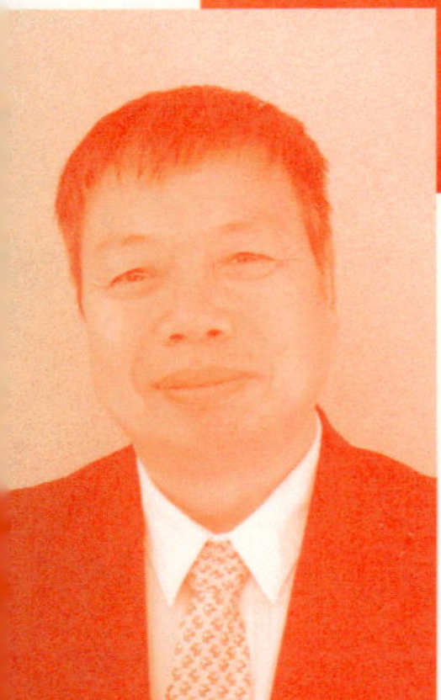
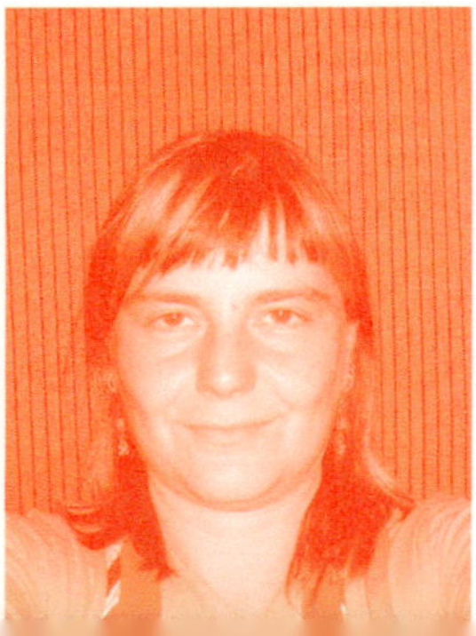

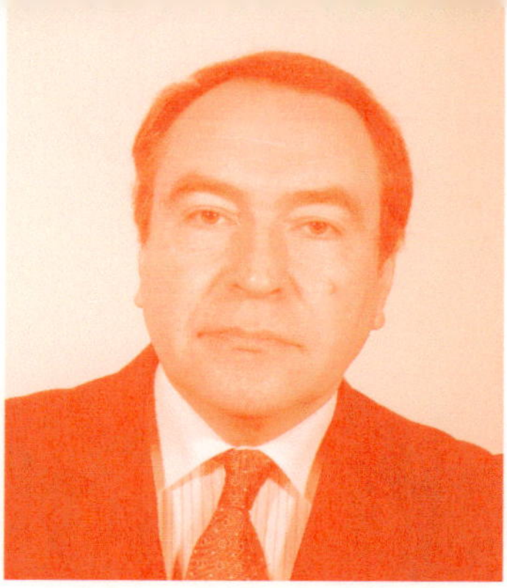

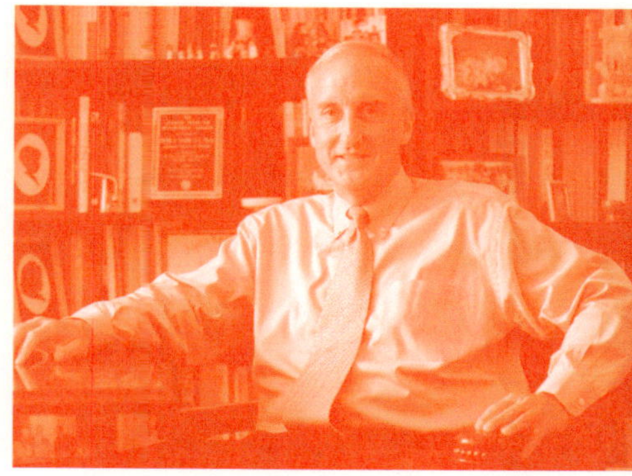

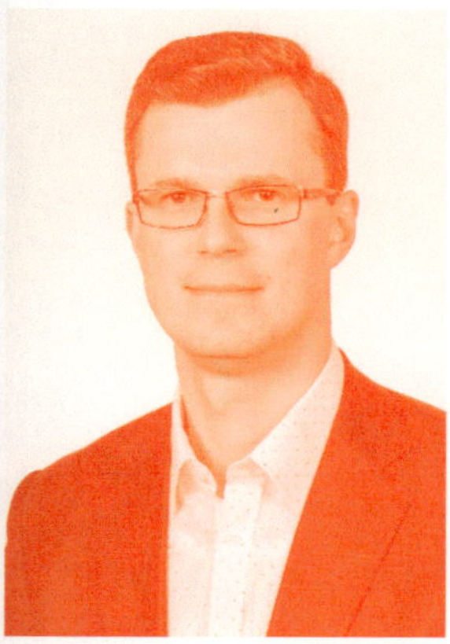

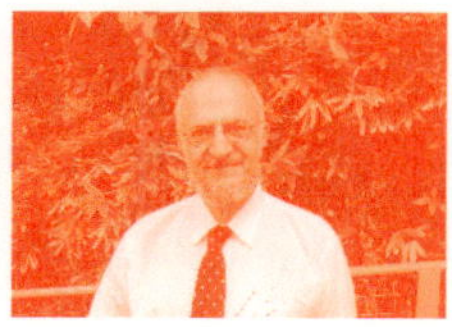

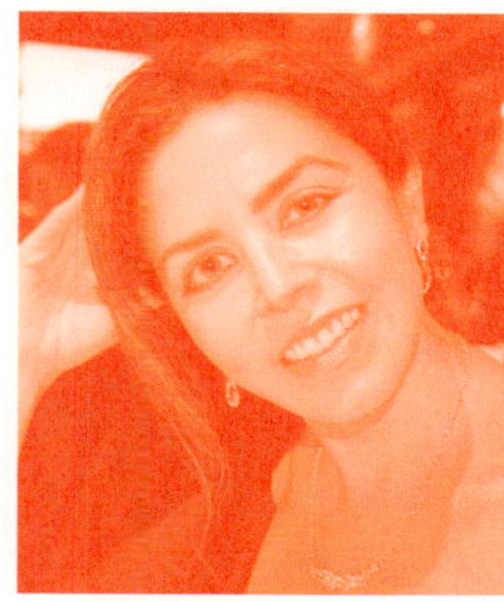

Supporting open minds since 2005

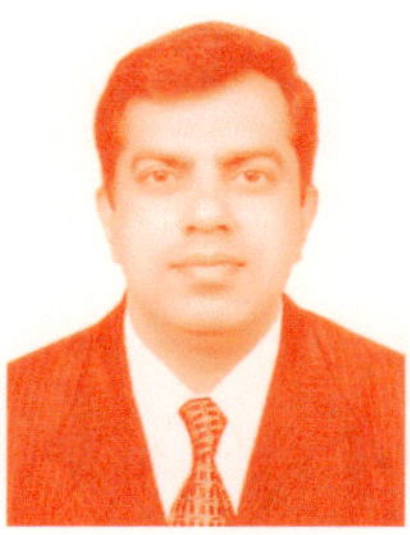

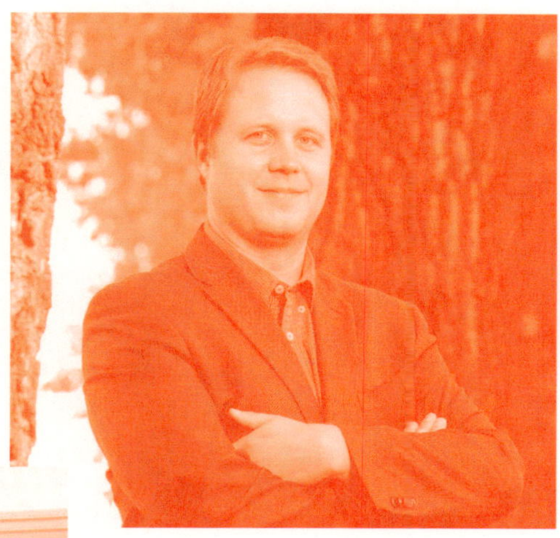

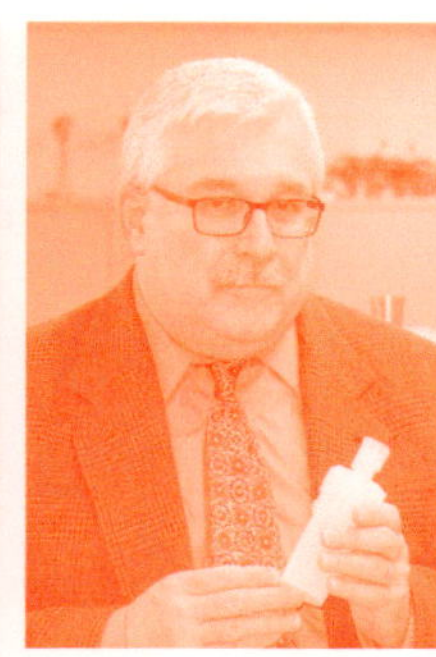

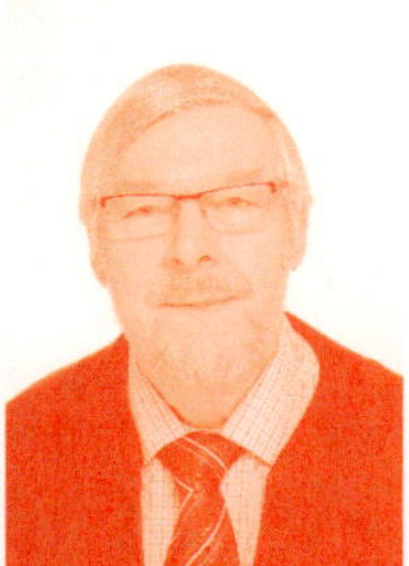

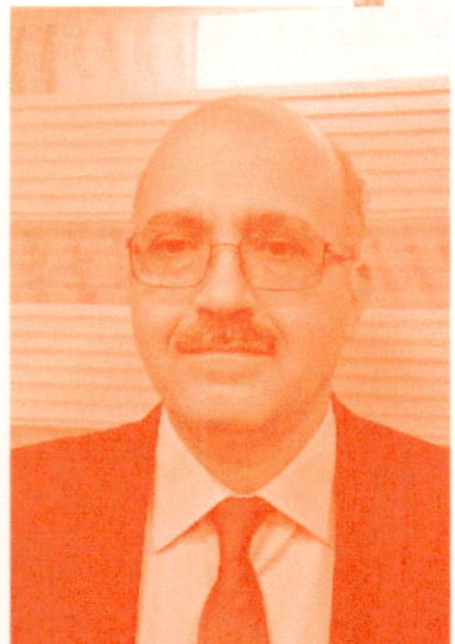

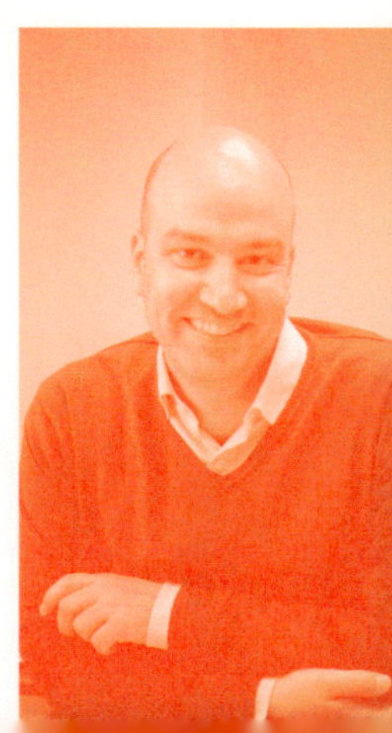

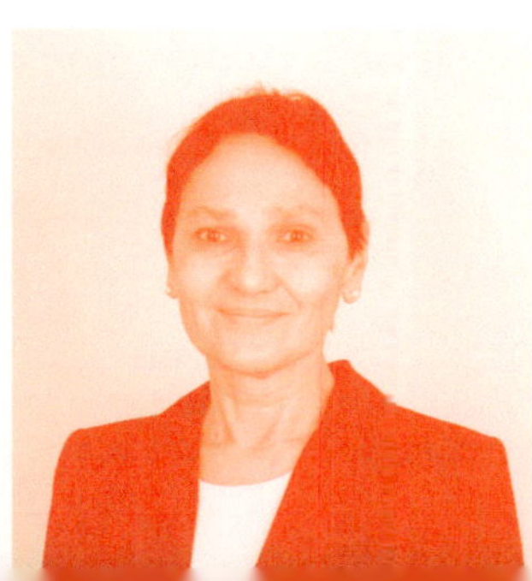

Periodontology - Fundamentals and Clinical Features
http://dx.doi.org/10.5772/intechopen.87277
Edited by Petra Surlin

Part of IntechOpen Book Series: Dentistry, Volume 8
Book Series Editor: Zühre Akarslan

Contributors
Silvia Martu, Irina-Georgeta Sufaru, Sorina-Mihaela Solomon, Ionut Luchian, Ioana Martu, Liliana Pasarin, Maria-Alexandra Martu, Monica-Silvia Tatarciuc, Dora-Maria Popescu, Elena Rezus, Diana Tatarciuc, Dorin Gheorghe, George-Alexandru Maftei, Sorina Mihaela Solomon, Liliana Georgeta Foia, Vasilica Toma, Shreya Kishore, Vanita Barai, Keerthi Venkatesan, Suvetha Siva, Juan Wu, Leung Wai Keung, Weibin Sun, Iulia Cristina Micu, Alexandra Roman, Andreea Ciurea, Gabriela Caracostea, Ada Delean, Marius Negucioiu, Dragos Alexandru Termure, Mircea Viorel Ciurea, Radu Chisnoiu, Adriana Objelean, Corina Ionescu, Alexandru Bucur, Andrada Soanca, Catalina Gabriela Pisoschi, Ana Marina Andrei, Elena Cristina Andrei, Elena Camelia Stănciulescu, Sandra Alice Buteică, Mihaela Cezarina Mehedinți, Ileana Monica Baniță, Mihaela Jana Țuculină, Subash Chandra Raj, Shaheda Tabassum, Annuroopa Mahapatra, Kaushik Patnaik, Santo Grace Umesh, Lakshmi Ramachandran, Janani Karthikeyan, Anitha Mani

Notice
Statements and opinions expressed in the chapters are these of the individual contributors and not necessarily those of the editors or publisher. No responsibility is accepted for the accuracy of information contained in the published chapters. The publisher assumes no responsibility for any damage or injury to persons or property arising out of the use of any materials, instructions, methods or ideas contained in the book.

First published in London, United Kingdom, 2022 by IntechOpen
IntechOpen is the global imprint of INTECHOPEN LIMITED, registered in England and Wales, registration number: 11086078, 5 Princes Gate Court, London, SW7 2QJ, United Kingdom
Printed in Croatia

British Library Cataloguing-in-Publication Data
A catalogue record for this book is available from the British Library

Additional hard and PDF copies can be obtained from orders@intechopen.com

Periodontology - Fundamentals and Clinical Features
Edited by Petra Surlin
p. cm.
Print ISBN 978-1-83880-678-1
Online ISBN 978-1-83880-679-8
eBook (PDF) ISBN 978-1-83880-680-4
ISSN 2631-6218

For EU product safety concerns:
IN TECH d.o.o., Prolaz Marije Krucifikse Kozulić 3, 51000 Rijeka, Croatia, info@intechopen.com or visit our website at intechopen.com.

IntechOpen Book Series
Dentistry
Volume 8

Prof. Petra Surlin, DMD, Ph.D., is a Professor of Periodontology at the University of Medicine and Pharmacy of Craiova, Romania. Following a periodontology specialization at the Universite Paris 7, Prof. Surlin became a consultant periodontology physician in 2012. The research work of Prof. Surlin is mainly focused on the field of periodontal medicine, specifically on the immunological interactions existing between periodontal disease and certain systemic conditions, like diabetes mellitus, rheumatoid arthritis, or hepatic diseases. The conducted research studies by Prof. Surlin, including research grants awarded by the Romanian Agency of Research and Innovation, have led to an extended publishing activity, comprising more than thirty Web of Science-indexed papers and over ten published books and book chapters with national and international publishing houses. Member of important professional associations, such as the European Federation of Periodontology (EFP) and the International Association of Dental Research (IADR), Prof. Surlin holds annual conferences and lectures at important dental and periodontology congresses and scientific meetings.

Editor of Volume 8: Petra Surlin
University of Medicine and Pharmacy of Craiova, Romania

Series Editor: Zühre Akarslan
Gazi University Faculty of Dentistry, Turkey

Scope of the Series

The major pathologies which dentists encounter in clinical practice include dental caries and periodontal diseases. Diagnosis and treatment of these pathologies is essential because when untreated, abscess could occur and it can even lead to the extraction of the tooth. Extracted teeth can be replaced with implants. Dentists and patients are nowadays more familiar with dental implant treatments. As a result, advanced diagnostic tools which aid in pre-operative treatment planning (cone-beam computed tomography, computer aided implant planning etc..), new implant designs improving the success of osteointegration, new materials, and techniques are introduced in the dental market.
Conditions which dentists frequently encounter in their clinical practice are temporomandibular joint (TMJ) disorders. These disorders include degenerative musculoskeletal conditions associated with morphological and functional deformities. Accurate diagnosis is important for proper management of TMJ pathologies. With

the advance in technology, new materials, techniques and equipment are introduced in the dental practice. New diagnostic aids in dental caries detection, cone-beam computed tomographic imaging, soft and hard tissue lasers, advances in oral and maxillofacial surgery procedures, uses of ultrasound, CAD/CAM, nanotechnology, plasma rich protein (PRP) and dental implantology are some of them. There will be even more new applications in dentistry in the future.

This book series includes topics related to dental caries, dentomaxillofacial imaging, new trends in oral implantology, new approaches in oral and maxillofacial surgery, temporomandibular joint disorders in dentistry etc.

Contents

Preface

This Edited Volume is a collection of reviewed and relevant research chapters, concerning the recent developments in periodontology. The book includes scholarly contributions by various authors and is edited by an expert pertinent to dental medicine. Each contribution comes as a separate chapter complete in itself but directly related to the book's topics and objectives.

The book is divided into 8 chapters. The target audience comprises scholars and specialists in the field.

IntechOpen

Chapter 1

Periodontal Medicine: Impact of Periodontal Status on Pregnancy Outcomes and Carcinogenesis

Gabriela Valentina Caracostea, Alexandru Bucur, Iulia Cristina Micu, Andrada Soanca, Andreea Ciurea, Adriana Objelean, Ada Gabriela Delean, Corina Violeta Ionescu, Radu Marcel Chisnoiu, Marius Negucioiu, Mircea Viorel Ciurea, Dragos Alexandru Termure and Alexandra Roman

Abstract

Periodontal medicine is a broad term commonly used to define the relationship between periodontitis and systemic health. Periodontitis is a highly prevalent, chronic multifactorial infectious disease, induced by the dysbiotic biofilm that triggers a persistent systemic inflammation and recurrent bacteremia. There is a growing body of scientific evidence that suggests the potential implication of periodontitis in the causation and progression of various systemic disease and conditions, such as diabetes, cardiovascular disease, pulmonary disease, adverse pregnancy outcomes and cancer. Some studies consider periodontitis as an independent risk factor for preterm birth, growth restriction, low birth-weight and pre-eclampsia. However not all studies support the association. Despite sparse scientific data, some studies indicate that individuals with periodontitis are at increased risk for cancer development, due to the increased inflammatory burden sustained by the presence of periodontal pathogens. This chapter emphasis the relationship between periodontitis and adverse pregnancy outcomes and the underlying mechanisms that link peridontitis to oral carcinogenesis.

Keywords: periodontitis, periodontal medicine, adverse pregnancy outcomes, preterm birth, malignancy, carcinogenesis, head, neck squamous cell carcinoma

1. Introduction

1.1 Periodontitis - overview

Periodontitis is a chronic disease, determined by the dysbiotic biofilm that does not merely affect the oral cavity, but also impacts the systemic health by triggering a persistent low-grade, systemic inflammation and recurrent bacteriemia. Its clinical consequences, especially in extended and severe forms, impair the overall quality of life of the individuals.

Significant progress has been made in determining the relationship between periodontitis and various systemic diseases. Some researchers consider periodontitis as an independent risk factor that mediates the development and even progression of certain systemic disease. Conversely, specific systemic diseases and conditions have a negative impact on the periodontium and can even interfere with periodontitis' progression. Valuable information are available with respect to several mechanisms underlying the correlation between periodontitis and systemic conditions. However, there are still plenty of issues, for which the scientific literature cannot currently provide specific answers, emphasizing their complexity and the need for further research in this area of interest.

1.2 Information search strategy and article selection

We conducted a search on the electronic database MEDLINE (PubMed) using MeSH terms and key words to identify relevant studies published between January 2011 and November 2020. One search strategy included the following subject terms combination: (["periodontitis"] OR ["periodontal disease"]) AND (["pregnancy outcome") OR ["preterm delivery"] OR ["birth weight"] OR ["pre-eclampsia"]). We searched another set of keywords as follows: (["periodontitis"]) OR ["periodontal disease"]) AND (["microbiota"] OR ["porphyromonas gingivalis"]) AND (["squamous cell carcinoma of head and neck"] OR ["head and neck neoplasms"] OR ["oropharyngeal neoplasms"] OR ["oral squamous cell carcinoma"] OR ["mouth neoplasms"]). Filters used were: Humans and English. A hand-search was also conducted to identify any additional related articles in Journal of Periodontology, Journal of Clinical Periodontology, and on the EFP Official Website/Gum disease & General Health Resources. Further articles of interest were searched based on reference lists of the publications where papers were available online. The presence of duplicates was assessed through Zotero version 5.0.93 software.

2. The periodontal medicine concept

Periodontitis is a highly prevalent, chronic multifactorial infectious disease, induced by the subgingival dysbiotic biofilm that produces a local immune-inflammatory response leading to the destruction of periodontal tissues. Its clinical manifestation, especially in extended and severe forms, impairs the overall quality of life, by affecting the psychosomatic, social and functional aspects of the individuals. Periodontitis also impacts the systemic health by triggering a persistent low-grade, systemic inflammation and recurrent bacteremia [1–4].

The concept of periodontal medicine was first introduced by Offenbacher [5]. Periodontal medicine is a broad term that describes an emerging branch of periodontology exploring the two way relationship between periodontal and systemic status, as well as new diagnostic tools and advanced treatment approaches that take into consideration the link between periodontitis and various systemic diseases [5]. Current evidence suggests that periodontitis acts as a biologically plausible risk factor for the development and progression of other chronic, inflammatory diseases [4].

Some associations between periodontitis and certain systemic conditions, such as diabetes mellitus, cardiovascular disease, and adverse pregnancy outcomes have been reported [6, 7]. However, there is still inconsistent information on the association between periodontitis and other systemic pathologies such as cancers, chronic renal disease, chronic obstructive pulmonary disease, minor cognitive impairment, rheumatoid arthritis, metabolic syndrome, and obesity [7, 8]. Contrarily, certain systemic diseases and conditions directly affect or worsen the periodontal status [9].

Establishing the potential causal relationship between periodontitis and chronic inflammatory systemic diseases and conditions is a difficult task, because complex pathologic conditions are the consequence of multiple exposures and broad interactions of external and host-derived factors that modulate disease initiation and development [1].

Noncommunicable diseases account for seven of ten worldwide deaths. In 2016, approximately 71% of the 56.9 million worldwide deaths were due to noncommunicable diseases and around 80% were due to cancers, cardiovascular diseases, chronic respiratory diseases and diabetes [10]. Since periodontitis is a potential, independent risk factor for many of these diseases, further investigations might bring additional benefits in improving the overall health status of the population and downsizing the socioeconomic burden at the same time.

3. Pathophysiological link between periodontitis and systemic diseases

Today there is increasing recognition that inflammation is a common molecular pathway that underlies the pathogenesis of diverse human diseases, ranging from infection to immune-mediated disorders, cardiovascular pathology, diabetes, metabolic syndrome, neurodegeneration, and cancer. Two pathogenic mechanisms might be involved in the activation of the pathways driving to development of pathologies at distant sites [11, 12].

The direct mechanism relies on the translocation of periodontal pathogens via systemic blood circulation, causing colonization and inflammation at a distance from the diseased periodontium. This mechanism corresponds to the concept of the "mobile oral microbiome" [13]. Moderate and severe periodontitis are characterized by deep periodontal pockets, with an ulcerated internal gingival epithelium, providing direct access for periodontal pathogens and their toxic by-products into the blood flow [12, 14]. Periodontal treatment, as well as daily tooth brushing cause episodic injuries to the periodontal tissues, which further leads to recurrent, transient bacteremia and endotoxinemia [11, 14]. On the other hand, bacterial and endotoxin dissemination may be enabled by macrophages and dendritic cells, serving as carriers for the pathogens [13, 15].

The indirect mechanism is defined by the systemic inflammatory response towards periodontal pathogens or as a result of metastatic periodontal inflammation [12, 13]. Systemic dissemination of periodontal pathogens triggers the activation of acute phase proteins in the liver, which amplify the systemic inflammatory response in order to provide protection against the bacterial threat. Acute phase protein production and the following events, as a response to periodontal infection, may affect the physiological functionality of other organs and systems. Moreover, cytokines play critical roles in orchestrating the effective immune response of leukocytes and parenchymal cells towards systemic bacteremia. Leukocytes are the major source of innate cytokine responses. A healthy immune system has the capacity to effectively eliminate pathogens and restore homeostasis. However, a dysfunctional immune response and an ineffective clearance will eventually lead to the initiation and progression of inflammatory diseases [11, 13, 14].

4. The relationship between periodontitis and pregnancy outcomes

4.1 The influence of hormonal variations in pregnancy on the periodontium

Pregnancy is characterized by significant fluctuations in the levels of progesterone and estrogen hormones reaching up to 30 times higher plasma levels, by the end of the third trimester. Various types of periodontal cells display receptors for these hormones [16, 17], which could explain the functional changes in the periodontal cells consecutive to fluctuating hormone levels during gestation, as well as microcirculatory system alterations [18]. These modifications are triggering an increased periodontal inflammatory manifestation, even in the presence of low levels of dental plaque, especially in the second and third trimesters of pregnancy. A gradual decrease of inflammatory manifestations after parturition has been reported [16–18].

Major alterations in the maternal immune system occur during pregnancy, which could favor periodontal infection and consecutive inflammation. Pregnant women have a reduction in phagocytosis and bactericidal activities of peripheral neutrophils and changes in the monocytes stimulated secretion of proinflammatory mediators after the contact with bacterial endotoxines [16].

Pregnancy not only impacts periodontal inflammation and host immune response, but also induces an increase in the oral microbial load and modifications in the oral microbiological profiles, as a consequence of elevated levels of steroid hormones [16, 18]. Significant changes in the subgingival microbiota with increases in the proportion of some periodontal pathogens such as *Bacteroides melaninogenicus*, *Prevotella intermedia*, and *Porphyromonas gingivalis* have been described [16].

Pregnancy increases the risk of new-onset periodontal disease, but it can also activate preexisting periodontitis leading to an infectious and inflammatory load similar to new-onset periodontitis. Maternal periodontitis may reflect an intrinsic inflammatory or innate immunity trait that places the woman at risk for severe forms of periodontal disease, as well as for the common terminal biochemical inflammatory cascade associated with adverse pregnancy outcomes [19].

4.2 Epidemiological associations between periodontitis and adverse pregnancy outcomes

Many studies have associated adverse pregnancy outcomes, such as low birth weight, preterm birth and preeclampsia, with maternal periodontitis. The first case–control study referring to the relationship between periodontitis and preterm-birth reported a 7.5 higher risk ratio for preterm births for the group of women with periodontitis as compared to the periodontal healthy control group [19]. Other studies have indicated oral maternal infections, including chronic periodontitis, as potential independent risk factors for various complications throughout the pregnancy. A systematic review including case–control, cohort case-control and controlled trials, confirmed the positive association between periodontitis and adverse pregnancy outcomes [20]. A meta-analysis reported a significant association between periodontitis and preterm birth, with an odds ratio of 1.38 [21]. A more recent meta-analyses including 10.215 women, indicates that periodontitis doubles the risk for preterm delivery, the calculated odds ratio being of 2.01 (95% CI 1.71–2.36) [22]. However, the level of association is mostly modest, mainly due to the high degree of heterogeneity between the studies, particularly with respect to the diversity of periodontitis disease case definitions [23].

The relationship between periodontitis and adverse pregnancy outcomes was investigated also by means of surrogate markers defining both conditions. Many studies indicate a positive association between gingival crevicular fluid, inflammatory mediators and adverse pregnancy outcomes [23, 24].

An umbrella review which analyzed systematic reviews and meta-analysis showed that non-surgical periodontal therapy with or without antibiotic therapy has low to moderate positive effects on reducing the frequency of the common pregnancy complications related to periodontitis [25]. The large heterogeneity of the outcomes of the interventional studies is due to variations in periodontitis case definition, sample particularities, follow-up period, control of confounding factors, as well as the therapy moment throughout the pregnancy [14, 25]. The nonsurgical periodontal therapy may be ineffective in reducing inflammatory cascade once activated and thus eventually lead to preterm birth [14].

4.3 Medical impact of adverse pregnancy outcomes

Preterm birth is defined as the birth prior to 37 weeks of gestation [26]. Complications of preterm birth are a leading cause of infant deaths worldwide raising the neonatal mortality risk rate up to 11.4 [27, 28]. The prevalence of preterm birth ranges from 5 to 7% in high-income countries, and is generally higher in low-income ones [29]. In 2014, the estimated global preterm birth rate was 10.6%, the equivalent of about 14.84 million preterm births from a total number of 139.95 million livebirths [30]. Therefore, prematurity is considered a major public health issue and the identification of any potential risk factor is of tremendous importance [27, 28, 30].

Low birth weight is defined as a birth weight below 2500 g regardless of gestational age of live infants [31, 32]. Various maternal factors such as extremes of maternal age, multiple pregnancies, obstetric complications, chronic maternal conditions like hypertensive disorders, and nutritional status or environmental exposures such as tobacco and drug use, can contribute to the low birth weight of the neonate. The estimates rate of global low birth weight for 2015 was 14.6% [31].

Maternal mortality is another important adverse outcome during pregnancy and is considered the death of a woman during pregnancy, within 42 days post-partum or during an abortion, as a consequence of any pregnancy associated pathological condition or complication [33]. The yearly number of global maternal deaths decreased from 532.000 in 1990, to 303.000 in 2015 [34]. Between 1990 and 2015, 10.7 million women worldwide died from various causes related to the evolution of pregnancy. Among the main risk factors of maternal mortality, pre-eclampsia and eclampsia are still in leading positions. Strategies aiming to reduce the number of deaths related to eclampsia showed a relatively low efficacy, which indicates the need to turn the attention to other potential risk factors in order to significantly lower mortality rates associated to eclampsia [33].

4.4 Pathophysiological link between periodontitis and adverse pregnancy outcomes

Hematogenous dissemination of periodontal bacteria is suspected to cause adverse pregnancy outcomes, by genitourinary tract and fetal–maternal unit colonization [16, 35]. Recent research indicates the presence of bacteria derived from supra- and subgingival biofilms in the placental microbiome. Moreover, some studies suggest that placental microbial profiles are closer to the oral microbial profiles than to the gut microbiome [36–38]. However, there is no general agreement on the bacterial translocation concept. The presence of oral bacteria in the placenta could be the consequence of an external contamination [39].

Although maternal infection is considered a major contributor of adverse pregnancy outcomes, a critical factor which can trigger the preterm birth might be rather the persistent inflammation generated by chronic periodontal infections. Inflammatory mediators that are abundantly produced at the affected sites determine periodontal tissue breakdown [14]. From a clinical point of view, deep periodontal pockets indicate the magnitude of the periodontal inflammation [39]. Chronic, long-term periodontal inflammation will eventually lead to a continuous passage of cytokines, chemokines, and gingival-derived C-reactive protein from the affected periodontal tissues into the bloodstream inducing a systemic acute-phase reaction and also maintaining a chronic, systemic inflammatory status [11, 12, 14]. High levels of C reactive protein over longer periods of time increases the risk for premature birth, but also of diabetes, and cardiovascular disease [13, 40].

Local and systemic accumulations of pro-inflammatory mediators, such as prostaglandins E2, interleukins, tumor necrosis factor α (TNF- α) and metalloproteinase (MMP) can stimulate the labor [41]. It is likely that spontaneous preterm parturition is induced by a high level of inflammation in the early stage of pregnancy [39]. However, the exact role of periodontal inflammation and the potential biological mechanisms that link periodontal disease with adverse pregnancy outcomes is not fully understood.

4.5 Clinical indications for pregnant women

European Federation of Periodontology guidelines for oral-health professionals provides the following recommendations [42]:

- During the examination of the oral status, dental professionals should always ask any female patient of childbearing age whether she is pregnant and should always consider pregnancy status before recommending any oral-health intervention.

- Inform women who are not pregnant of the importance of oral and periodontal health during pregnancy and of the treatment of existing periodontal diseases before becoming pregnant.

- For any pregnant women, perform a comprehensive clinical periodontal examination and formulate a diagnosis of “healthy”, “gingivitis”, or “periodontitis”.

- Pregnant women with a healthy periodontium should be provided with oral-health education and preventive personal plaque control measures that should became healthy habits throughout life. Also, provide information on the inflammatory periodontal events that could occur during pregnancy (increased gingival bleeding and gingival enlargement).

- Pregnant woman with gingivitis should be provided with the same oral-health education and personal plaque control measures, as well as professional mechanical instrumentation for removing plaque and calculus deposits from the tooth surfaces. The reevaluation of the periodontal status, in terms of efficacy of the professional and personal interventions and periodontal monitoring throughout pregnancy are mandatory.

- Pregnant women with periodontitis should also have the same oral-health educational measures, as well as additional professional intervention by means of standard non-surgical periodontal therapy (scaling and root planing).

- Non-surgical periodontal therapy, dental treatments and extractions are safe during pregnancy, mainly during the second trimester of gestation.

- Local anesthesia, common painkillers and systemic antibiotics are generally safe without additional risk to the foetus or the pregnant woman.

- Tetracyclines should be strictly avoided. Other medication should be prescribed to the pregnant woman after communication with her obstetrician.

- Although EFP recommends dental x-rays and chemical plaque-control agents during pregnancy, the authors of the present chapter are not keen to recommending them.

5. Implications of periodontitis in oral carcinogenesis

5.1 Epidemiological associations between periodontitis and head and neck squamos cell carcinoma

Cancer is one of the leading causes of worldwide mortality. In 2016, 1.1 million new cases were reported, and the prevalence was of 4.1 million cases. Head and neck squamous cell carcinomas (HNSCCs) constituted 5.7% of global cancer-related mortality, the equivalent of 512.770 deaths. Also the global mortality burden is expected to increase; by 2030 an estimated 705.902 people worldwide will be expected to die due to HNSCC [43]. This great burden of cancer worldwide strongly indicates the need for implementing rigorous screening and control programs in order to facilitate the identification of all potential HNSCC related risk factors, including periodontitis, and the early detection of HNSCC.

Squamous cell carcinoma is the most common histological subtype of oral and oropharyngeal malignant tumors, accounting for about 90% of the cases. The incidence of HNSCCs are reported to be on the rise, with a global estimated incidence of over 300.000 new cases registered each year [44, 45].

Emerging evidence indicates periodontitis as a potential independent risk factor for the development of premalignant lesions and HNSCC [46, 47]. Current evidence regarding a positive association between periodontitis and oral and oropharyngeal cancers are currently controversial [48]. Some studies suggest an increased susceptibility to HNSCC in periodontitis patients [49]. Extended and severe forms of periodontitis have been frequently identified among patients with HNSCC [48].

A meta-analysis reported a 2.66-fold higher risk for oral cancer in patients with periodontal disease as compared to periodontal healthy controls [50]. A hospital-based case-cohort study, after controlling for important confounders, found that individuals with periodontitis were 3.7 times more likely to have oral squamous cell carcinoma as compared to individuals without periodontitis [51].

Positive associations between periodontitis and other cancers such as digestive tract cancer, pancreatic cancer, prostate cancer, breast cancer, corpus uteri cancer, lung cancer, hematological cancer, and Non-Hodgkin lymphoma have been reported [46].

The relationship between periodontitis and HNSCC has been reported based on the specific periodontal parameters or surrogate markers of periodontal disease. An increased risk of HNSCC development, with respect to the number of missing teeth has been observed. A 2.7-fold increased risk of oral cancer in patients having 11 to 16 missing teeth as compared to dentate subjects has been reported [52]. A 5.23-fold increase in the risk of tongue cancer and a 4-fold increased risk of head and neck squamous cell carcinoma for each millimeter of alveolar bone loss, after the adjustment for important confounders has been reported [53, 54]. This data suggest that the severity and extension of periodontitis might be a risk indicator for HNSCC [55].

5.2 The influence of chronic periodontal inflammation in carcinogenesis

The investigation of the causal role of periodontitis in the cancer development is challenging due to the major independent and shared risk factors of these conditions. Periodontitis may have a direct effect on the rise of cancer risk or may impact through shared genetic and environmental factors [56]. Smoking is one of the main independent risk factors for periodontitis and HNSCC, while smoking and alcohol consumptions account for up to 85% of all oral cancers. The synergic effect of alcohol and tobacco consumption increases the risk for of oral cancer by 15 times [57, 58] However, about 15% to 20% of the HNSCCs occur independently to any of these risk factors, and the clinical features and evolution of the cancer in this group is often particularly aggressive [57–60].

Some molecular pathogenic mechanism could associate periodontitis to oral cancers and are briefly detailed below.

5.2.1 Destruction of epithelial barrier promotes the passage of toxic compounds

Chronic periodontal inflammation might be an extrinsic pathway in cancer development [46, 47, 61, 62]. The damage of the junctional epithelium mediated by periodontal pathogens alters its protective function promoting the absorption of toxic compounds from alcohol and tobacco, which in turn create a chronic inflammatory environment [61, 63]. The inflammatory process and the presence of cell-stimulating signals may create an optimal environment for the atypical cell proliferation and differentiation, which may eventually lead to cancer development [46, 61, 63].

5.2.2 Increased pro-inflammatory periodontal mediators damage DNA

In periodontitis, the complex inflammatory response developed to eliminate periodontal pathogens leads to the accumulation of excessive levels of endogenous compounds such as cytokines, chemokines, prostaglandins, reactive oxygen and nitrogen species, matrix metalloproteinases, and endothelial and epidermal growth factors. The anarchic and excessive release of these molecules is responsible for the indirect destruction of periodontal tissues [64]. In the meantime, these proinflammatory molecules may irreversibly damage the cellular DNA, deregulate the mechanisms of DNA repair and subvert the cell cycle regulatory mechanisms [65, 66]. Thus, cumulative, permanent genetic alterations lead to oncogenes activation or tumor suppressor genes inactivation [67].

5.2.3 Increased proinflammatory periodontal mediators promote epigenetic modifications

Epigenetic changes occur more frequently than gene mutations and may persist for the entire cell life and even for multiple generations. Extensive exposure of oral mucosa to bacteria and chemokines may contribute to carcinogenesis by causing epigenetic alterations. The epigenetic changes, which refer to any heritable modifications in gene expression without alterations of the DNA sequence, also promote genomic instability. Epigenetic mechanisms include DNA methylation, posttranslational modifications of histone proteins and post-transcriptional gene down-regulation by microRNAs. Any of these three distinct epigenetic mechanisms leads to inappropriate gene expression and cancer development [61, 67, 68]. A relatively stable epigenetic change may induce the increase of carcinogenesis mechanisms such as faster cellular proliferation, stimulation of an increased angiogenesis, and inhibition of apoptosis [61].

The methylation of DNA refers to the covalent addition of a methyl group to the 5-carbon position of cytosine base from a CpG dinucleotide. Hypermetilation of CpG islands of growth-regulatory genes promoter regions causes the transcriptional "silencing" of tumor suppressor genes and promotes tumor progression [68]. Although some aberrant methylation patterns have been already identified, the complex underlying molecular mechanisms that address the association of chronic periodontal inflammation and oral cancers are still not fully understood [61].

Histones, proteins binding to the DNA in the nucleus and condensing it into chromatin, can undergo multiple aberrant post-translational modifications, which induce structural and functional modification in the chromatin and thus alterations of the pattern of gene expression directly contributing to the initiation of neoplasia and its subsequent course [68].

5.2.4 The increased release of pro-inflammatory mediators

The increased release of inflammatory mediators in periodontitis, such as interleukin-6 (IL-6), interleukin-8 (IL-8), and tumor necrosis factor–α (TNF–α) [61], may trigger epithelial-mesenchymal transition and activation of inflammatory cells which facilitate cancer invasion [61, 69].

5.2.5 Increased levels of IL-8 regulate carcinoma growth

IL-8 is primarily produced by periodontal cells in response to periodontal bacteria, like *Porphyromonas gingivalis*, and bacterial toxins [13, 70]. One of the possible links between *Porphyromonas gingivalis* and oral squamous cell carcinoma may be the increased IL-8 levels in the periodontal microenvironment and the subsequent overexpression of MMPs. IL-8 has long been recognized as an autocrine regulator of oral squamos cell carcinoma growth, and a contributor of increased cell motility. Thus, salivary IL-8 has been proposed to be a discriminative diagnostic biomarker for oral cancer detection [69, 70].

5.2.6 The influence of inflammasomes-mediated inflammation in cancer

More recent studies investigated the topic of inflammasome-mediated inflammation in cancer. The inflammasome is a part of the innate immune system and it responds to microbial challenge through regulation of caspase-1 activation and induction of inflammation. The most studied and best characterized inflammasome, Nucleotide-Binding Domain, Leucine-Rich–Containing Family, Pyrin Domain–Containing-3 (NLRP3), is an emerging, key player in the development and progression of cancer. Activation of NLRP3 may promote inflammation induced tumor growth and metastasis in HNSCC [71]. Certain periodontal pathogens, such as *Porphyromonas gingivalis* and *Aggregatibacter actinomycetemcomitans* have the ability to modulate inflammation and potentially induce carcinogenesis by controlling interleukin-1β (IL-1β) secretion through NRLP3 inflammasome complex activated by adenosine 5 '- triphosphate (ATP). IL-1β is directly involved in several chronic pathologies and various types of cancers, including oral cancer [72, 73].

5.2.7 The role of transcription factors

Inflammatory mediators, microbes, as well as environmental factors (tobacco and alcohol consumption) could activate some transcription factors, such as the nuclear signal transducers and activators of transcription-3 (STAT-3), the activator protein-1 (AP-1) and the nuclear factor-kB (NF-kB). These transcription factors activate oncogenes that regulate apoptosis, cell proliferation and angiogenesis as well as genes regulating the production of pro-inflammatory molecules. These oncogenic changes drive a tumor-promoting inflammatory milieu through the intrinsic pathway that favors the development of already established tumors. Moreover, the inflammatory microenvironment favors the tumor to escape from immune surveillance and alters the response to chemotherapy [65, 66, 74].

5.2.8 Periodontitis associated-oxidative stress promoting carcinogenesis

Oxidative stress occurs as a state of disturbance between free radical production and the capability of antioxidant system to counteract the free radicals. The activity of periodontal bacteria induces oxidative stress through free radical release, and decreased plasma antioxidant capacity. On the other hand, oxidative stress causes inflammation, which can increase the production of free radicals. Patients with chronic periodontitis showed low serum and salivary antioxidants levels and elevated oxidative stress biomarkers such as 8-isoprostane and malondialdehyde. Moreover, assessment of blood and gingival tissues of chronic periodontitis patients also revealed mitochondrial DNA deletion mediated by lipid peroxidation [73].

Oxidative stress is also correlated to oral cancer. Increased lipid peroxidation and reduced antioxidants was reported in patients with oral cancer. Lipid peroxidation and irreversible protein modifications are essential molecular mechanisms involved in the oxidative damage of cell structures eventually leading to programmed cell death [73, 75]. Elevated levels of malondialdehyde and low levels of glutathione were observed in the saliva and serum of HNSCC patients [73, 76].

Chronic periodontal inflammation induces a prolonged exposure of oral cells to free radicals that can lead to genomic alterations through DNA damage, lipid and protein peroxidation and activation of signal transduction by post translational modification [66]. Therefore, the accumulation of oxidative stress products in periodontal tissues may significantly contribute to the development of oral cancer.

Oncogene and tumor suppressor pathways are proven intracellular targets for therapies, but recent scientific data are pointing out to new potential, *extracellular* vesicle-based therapeutic targets such as chemokines and chemokines receptors. Anti-inflammatory therapies have been successful in preventing progression and even curing some types of infectious agents associated cancers [66, 74]. Hence, control of chronic periodontal inflammation through specific periodontal therapy could be part of a comprehensive HNSCCs prevention strategy.

5.3 Periodontal bacteria in carciongenesis - *Porphyromona gingivalis*

Porphyromonas gingivalis is a true periodontal pathogen contributing in development of severe chronic inflammations of periodontal tissues. *Porphyromonas gingivalis* has been frequently associate with cancer and the most highly associated organism with oral squamous cell carcinomas [72]. Besides colonizing dental surfaces, the microorganism is also able to colonize various parts of the oral mucosa, which are described to be primary lesion sites during oral squamous cell cancer initiation [72].

Porphyromonas gingivalis produces various virulence factors which can modulate oral persistent inflammation and thus the complex physio-pathological network leading to carcinogenesis [72, 77]. *Porphyromonas gingivalis* as well as other periodontal microorganisms can trigger the development of a dysbiotic microbhabitat. *Porphyromonas gingivalis* has the capacity of disrupting the periodontal homeostasis by promoting the transformation of the commensal microbiota into a pathological one. Also it can modulate the host's immune system, thus being able to intervene directly in the development of cancers at the oral or distant sites [78].

Porphyromonas gingivalis invades oral epithelial cells and could affect cell cycle related molecules at different stages [79]. Epithelial cell responses to *Porphyromonas gingivalis* infection include both changes to apoptosis and cell division [72, 77, 79]; these mechanisms are characteristic to cancer development and progression.

Porphyromonas gingivalis lipopolysaccharides could deregulate tumor suppressor gene p53 [72, 77]. Gingipains and cysteine proteinases produced by *Porphyromonas gingivalis*, play a key role in activating MMP-9, which degrades the basement membrane and the extracellular matrix, promoting carcinoma cell migration and invasion, thus allowing dissemination and metastatic growth at remote sites [72, 77, 78, 80]. Also in oral squamous cell carcinoma cells, *Porphyromonas gingivalis* stimulates the release of a variety of cytokines, including IL-8, which can increase MMP-9 production and cell proliferation and invasiveness [80].

Porphyromonas gingivalis can also modulate the expression of microRNAs of the epithelial cells, and up-regulation of miR-203 leads to inhibition of the negative regulator suppressor of cytokine signaling 3 and subsequent suppression of apoptosis [77].

Porphyromonas gingivalis secretes a nucleoside diphosphate kinase (NDK) having an ATPase function and preventing ATP-dependent apoptosis mediated through the purinergic receptor P2X7. Thus, NDK can suppress the proapoptotic and proinflammatory mechanisms in oral epithelial cells favoring carcinogenesis [72, 77].

The heat shock protein GroEL is another virulence factor of *Porphyromonas gingivalis* that might have a direct carcinogenic effects on certain oral cancer cell lines [72].

Porphyromonas gingivalis can induce the expression of the B7-H1 and B7-DC involved in regulating the cell-mediated immune response, but also up-regulated in cells originating from a variety of cancers. B7-H1 expression promotes the event of regulatory T cells that suppress effector T cells. B7-H1 expression might contribute to immune evasion by oral cancers [47, 77, 80].

Currently, among the known virulence molecules of *Porphyromonas gingivalis*, there is not a significantly attributed molecular determinant that could be strongly linked to the illustrated association of *Porphyromonas gingivalis* with orodigestive cancers. It is very likely that the potential synergistic ability of *Porphyromonas gingivalis* with other oral microbial species are contributory to the postulated malignant transformation and progression in the oral cavity and upper digestive tract [72].

6. Conclusions

Understanding the dynamics and common, underlying pathophysiological mechanisms that link periodontitis to systemic diseases is essential to the development of coherent, patient centered diagnostic and therapeutic strategies.

An increased risk for preterm birth and low birth weight of newborns in mothers with periodontitis has been reported. Pregnant women should be provided with oral-health education and preventive personal plaque control measures that should become healthy habits throughout life. Non-surgical periodontal therapy is safe during pregnancy, and especially during the second trimester of gestation.

The epigenetic alterations in periodontal disease such as histone acetylation and DNA methylation, and the subsequently altered gene expression might partially explain the role of periodontal inflammation in cancer development and tumor growth.

Conflict of interest

The authors declare no conflict of interest.

Author details

Gabriela Valentina Caracostea[1], Alexandru Bucur[2], Iulia Cristina Micu[3*], Andrada Soanca[4], Andreea Ciurea[3], Adriana Objelean[5], Ada Gabriela Delean[6], Corina Violeta Ionescu[6], Radu Marcel Chisnoiu[6], Marius Negucioiu[7], Mircea Viorel Ciurea[8], Dragos Alexandru Termure[8] and Alexandra Roman[4]

1 Department of Obstetrics and Gynecology, Faculty of Medicine, "Iuliu Hatieganu" University of Medicine and Pharmacy, Emergency County Clinical Hospital, Cluj-Napoca, Romania

2 Department of Oro-Maxillo-Facial Surgery, Faculty of Dental Medicine, "Carol Davila" University of Medicine and Pharmacy, "Prof. Dr. Dan Theodorescu" Oro-Maxillo-Facial Clinical Hospital, Bucharest, Romania

3 Department of Periodontology, Faculty of Dental Medicine, "Iuliu Hatieganu" University of Medicine and Pharmacy, Cluj-Napoca, Romania

4 Department of Periodontology, Faculty of Dental Medicine, "Iuliu Hatieganu" University of Medicine and Pharmacy, Emergency County Clinical Hospital, Cluj-Napoca, Romania

5 Department of Dental Materials and Ergonomics, Faculty of Dental Medicine, "Iuliu Hatieganu" University of Medicine and Pharmacy, Cluj-Napoca, Romania

6 Department of Conservative Odontology, Faculty of Dental Medicine, "Iuliu Hatieganu" University of Medicine and Pharmacy, Cluj-Napoca, Romania

7 Department of Prosthetic Dentistry, Faculty of Dental Medicine, "Iuliu Hatieganu" University of Medicine and Pharmacy, Emergency County Clinical Hospital, Cluj-Napoca, Romania

8 Department of Oral and Maxillofacial Surgery, Faculty of Dental Medicine, "Iuliu Hatieganu" University of Medicine and Pharmacy, Cluj-Napoca, Romania

*Address all correspondence to: i.cristina.micu@gmail.com

References

[1] Chapple IL. Time to take periodontitis seriously. BMJ. 2014;348:g2645. DOI:10.1136/bmj.g2645. DOI: 10.1136/bmj.g2645

[2] Ferreira MC, Dias-Pereira AC, Branco-de-Almeida LS, Martins CC, Paiva SM. Impact of periodontal disease on quality of life: a systematic review. J Periodontal Res. 2017;52(4):651-665. DOI:10.1111/jre.12436

[3] Peres MA, Macpherson LMD, Weyant RJ, Daly B, Venturelli R, Mathur MR, et al. Oral diseases: a global public health challenge [published correction appears in Lancet. 2019;394(10203):1010]. Lancet. 2019;394(10194):249-260. doi:10.1016/S0140-6736(19)31146-8

[4] Papapanou PN, Susin C. Periodontitis epidemiology: is periodontitis under-recognized, over-diagnosed, or both?. Periodontol 2000. 2017;75(1):45-51. DOI:10.1111/prd.12200

[5] Offenbacher S. Periodontal diseases: pathogenesis. Ann Periodontol. 1996;1(1):821-878. DOI:10.1902/annals.1996.1.1.821

[6] Beck JD, Offenbacher S. The association between periodontal diseases and cardiovascular diseases: a state-of-the-science review. Ann Periodontol. 2001;6(1):9-15. DOI:10.1902/annals.2001.6.1.9

[7] Monsarrat P, Blaizot A, Kémoun P, Ravaud P, Nabet C, Sixou M, et al. Clinical research activity in periodontal medicine: a systematic mapping of trial registers. J Clin Periodontol. 2016;43(5):390-400. DOI:10.1111/jcpe.12534

[8] Linden GJ, Herzberg MC; Working group 4 of joint EFP/AAP workshop. Periodontitis and systemic diseases: a record of discussions of working group 4 of the Joint EFP/AAP Workshop on Periodontitis and Systemic Diseases. J Clin Periodontol. 2013;40 Suppl 14:S20-S23. DOI:10.1111/jcpe.12091

[9] Williams RC, Offenbacher S. Periodontal medicine: the emergence of a new branch of periodontology. Periodontol 2000. 2000;23:9-12. DOI:10.1034/j.1600-0757.2000.2230101.x

[10] NCD Countdown 2030 collaborators. NCD Countdown 2030: worldwide trends in non-communicable disease mortality and progress towards Sustainable Development Goal target 3.4. Lancet. 2018;392(10152):1072-1088. DOI:10.1016/S0140-6736(18)31992-5

[11] Kornman KS. Contemporary approaches for identifying individual risk for periodontitis. Periodontol 2000. 2018;78(1):12-29. DOI:10.1111/prd.12234

[12] Winning L, Linden GJ. Periodontitis and Systemic Disease: Association or Causality?. Curr Oral Health Rep. 2017;4(1):1-7. DOI:10.1007/s40496-017-0121-7

[13] Hasturk H, Kantarci A. Activation and resolution of periodontal inflammation and its systemic impact. Periodontol 2000. 2015;69(1):255-273. DOI:10.1111/prd.12105

[14] Papapanou PN. Systemic effects of periodontitis: lessons learned from research on atherosclerotic vascular disease and adverse pregnancy outcomes. Int Dent J. 2015;65(6):283-291. DOI:10.1111/idj.12185

[15] Hajishengallis G. Periodontitis: from microbial immune subversion to systemic inflammation. Nat Rev Immunol. 2015;15(1):30-44. DOI:10.1038/nri3785

[16] Armitage GC. Bi-directional relationship between pregnancy and periodontal disease. Periodontol 2000. 2013;61(1):160-176. DOI:10.1111/j.1600-0757.2011.00396.x

[17] Bobetsis YA, Graziani F, Gürsoy M, Madianos PN. Periodontal disease and adverse pregnancy outcomes. Periodontol 2000. 2020;83(1):154-174. DOI:10.1111/prd.12294

[18] Silva de Araujo Figueiredo C, Gonçalves Carvalho Rosalem C, Costa Cantanhede AL, Abreu Fonseca Thomaz ÉB, Fontoura Nogueira da Cruz MC. Systemic alterations and their oral manifestations in pregnant women. J Obstet Gynaecol Res. 2017;43(1):16-22. DOI:10.1111/jog.13150

[19] Offenbacher S, Boggess KA, Murtha AP, Jared HL, Lieff S, McKaig RG, et al. Progressive periodontal disease and risk of very preterm delivery Obstet Gynecol. 2006;107(1):29-36. DOI:10.1097/01.AOG.0000190212.87012.96

[20] Xiong X, Buekens P, Fraser WD, Beck J, Offenbacher S. Periodontal disease and adverse pregnancy outcomes: a systematic review. BJOG. 2006;113(2):135-143. DOI:10.1111/j.1471-0528.2005.00827.x

[21] Petrini M, Gursoy M, Gennai S, Graziani F. Biological mechanisms between periodontal diseases and pregnancy complications: a systematic review and meta-analysis of epidemiological association between adverse pregnancy outcomes and periodontitis - an update of the review by Ide & Papapanou (2013). Eur Fed Periodontol. 2017. Availabe from:https://www.efp.org/publications/projects/oralhealthandpregnancy/reports/review-biological-mechanisms.html. [Accessed 17-11-2020]

[22] Manrique-Corredor EJ, Orozco-Beltran D, Lopez-Pineda A, Quesada JA, Gil-Guillen VF, Carratala-Munuera C. Maternal periodontitis and preterm birth: Systematic review and meta-analysis. Community Dent Oral Epidemiol. 2019;47(3):243-251. DOI:10.1111/cdoe.12450

[23] Sanz M, Kornman K; working group 3 of the joint EFP/AAP workshop. Periodontitis and adverse pregnancy outcomes: consensus report of the Joint EFP/AAP Workshop on Periodontitis and Systemic Diseases. J Periodontol. 2013;84(4 Suppl):S164-S169. DOI:10.1902/jop.2013.1340016

[24] Stadelmann P, Alessandri R, Eick S, Salvi GE, Surbek D, Sculean A. The potential association between gingival crevicular fluid inflammatory mediators and adverse pregnancy outcomes: a systematic review. Clin Oral Investig. 2013;17(6):1453-1463. DOI: 10.1007/s00784-013-0952-0

[25] Rangel-Rincón LJ, Vivares-Builes AM, Botero JE, Agudelo-Suárez AA. An Umbrella Review Exploring the Effect of Periodontal Treatment in Pregnant Women on the Frequency of Adverse Obstetric Outcomes. J Evid Based Dent Pract. 2018;18(3):218-239. DOI:10.1016/j.jebdp.2017.10.0 11s00784-013-0952-0

[26] ACOG Committee Opinion No 579: Definition of term pregnancy. Obstet Gynecol. 2013;122(5):1139-1140. DOI:10.1097/01.AOG.0000437385.88715.4a

[27] Leviton A, Paneth N, Reuss ML, Susser M, Allred EN, Dammann O, et al. Maternal infection, fetal inflammatory response, and brain damage in very low birth weight infants. Developmental Epidemiology Network Investigators. Pediatr Res. 1999;46(5):566-575. DOI:10.1203/00006450-199911000-00013

[28] Ward RM, Beachy JC. Neonatal complications following preterm

birth. BJOG. 2003;110 Suppl 20:8-16. DOI:10.1016/s1470-0328(03)00012-0

[29] Beck S, Wojdyla D, Say L, Betran AP, Merialdi M, Requejo JH, et al. The worldwide incidence of preterm birth: a systematic review of maternal mortality and morbidity. Bull World Health Organ. 2010;88(1):31-38. doi:10.2471/BLT.08.062554

[30] Chawanpaiboon S, Vogel JP, Moller AB, Lumbiganon P, Petzold M, Hogan D, et al. Global, regional, and national estimates of levels of preterm birth in 2014: a systematic review and modelling analysis. Lancet Glob Health. 2019;7(1):e37-e46. DOI:10.1016/S2214-109X(18)30451-0

[31] Blencowe H, Krasevec J, de Onis M, Black RE, An X, Stevens GA, et al. National, regional, and worldwide estimates of low birthweight in 2015, with trends from 2000: a systematic analysis. Lancet Glob Health. 2019;7(7):e849-e860. DOI:10.1016/S2214-109X(18)30565-5

[32] Konopka T, Paradowska-Stolarz A. Periodontitis and risk of preterm birth and low birthweight--a meta-analysis. Ginekol Pol. 2012;83(6):446-453

[33] Say L, Chou D, Gemmill A, Tunçalp Ö, Moller A-B, Daniels J, et al. Global causes of maternal death: a WHO systematic analysis. Lancet Glob Health. 2014;2(6):e323-e333. DOI:10.1016/S2214-109X(14)70227-X

[34] Alkema L, Chou D, Hogan D, Zhang S, Moller A-B, Gemmill A, et al.Global, regional, and national levels and trends in maternal mortality between 1990 and 2015, with scenario-based projections to 2030: a systematic analysis by the UN Maternal Mortality Estimation Inter-Agency Group. Lancet. 2016;387(10017):462-474. DOI:10.1016/S0140-6736(15)00838-7

[35] Vander Haar EL, So J, Gyamfi-Bannerman C, Han YW. Fusobacterium nucleatum and adverse pregnancy outcomes: Epidemiological and mechanistic evidence. Anaerobe. 2018;50:55-59. doi:10.1016/j.anaerobe.2018.01.008

[36] Aagaard K, Ma J, Antony KM, Ganu R, Petrosino J, Versalovic J. The placenta harbors a unique microbiome. Sci Transl Med. 2014;6(237):237ra65. DOI:10.1126/scitranslmed.3008599

[37] Chopra A, Radhakrishnan R, Sharma M. *Porphyromonas gingivalis* and adverse pregnancy outcomes: a review on its intricate pathogenic mechanisms. *Crit Rev Microbiol*. 2020;46(2):213-236. DOI:10.1080/1040841X.2020.1747392

[38] Han YW. Fusobacterium nucleatum: a commensal-turned pathogen. Curr Opin Microbiol. 2015;23:141-147. DOI:10.1016/j.mib.2014.11.013

[39] Fischer LA, Demerath E, Bittner-Eddy P, Costalonga M. Placental colonization with periodontal pathogens: the potential missing link. Am J Obstet Gynecol. 2019;221(5):383-392.e3.DOI:10.1016/j.ajog.2019.04.029

[40] Pitiphat W, Joshipura KJ, Rich-Edwards JW, Williams PL, Douglass CW, Gillman MW. Periodontitis and plasma C-reactive protein during pregnancy. J Periodontol. 2006;77(5):821-825. DOI:10.1902/jop.2006.050193

[41] Al Habashneh R, Khader YS, Jabali OA, Alchalabi H. Prediction of preterm and low birth weight delivery by maternal periodontal parameters: receiver operating characteristic (ROC) curve analysis. Matern Child Health J. 2013;17(2):299-306. DOI:10.1007/s10995-012-0974-2

[42] Resources - Categories: Guidelines. European Federation of Periodontology. 2020. Available from: https://www.efp.org/gum-disease-general-health/

oral-health-pregnancy/resources/guidelines/ [Accessed 17-11-2020]

[43] Patterson RH, Fischman VG, Wasserman I, Siu J, Shrime MG, Fagan JJ, et al. Global Burden of Head and Neck Cancer: Economic Consequences, Health, and the Role of Surgery. Otolaryngol Head Neck Surg. 2020;162(3):296-303. DOI:10.1177/0194599819897265

[44] Chi AC, Day TA, Neville BW. Oral cavity and oropharyngeal squamous cell carcinoma--an update. CA Cancer J Clin. 2015;65(5):401-421. doi:10.3322/caac.21293

[45] Thomson PJ. Perspectives on oral squamous cell carcinoma prevention-proliferation, position, progression and prediction. J Oral Pathol Med. 2018;47(9):803-807. DOI:10.1111/jop.12733

[46] Corbella S, Veronesi P, Galimberti V, Weinstein R, Del Fabbro M, Francetti L. Is periodontitis a risk indicator for cancer? A meta-analysis. PLoS One. 2018;13(4):e0195683. DOI:10.1371/journal.pone.0195683

[47] Gholizadeh P, Eslami H, Yousefi M, Asgharzadeh M, Aghazadeh M, Kafil HS. Role of oral microbiome on oral cancers, a review. Biomed Pharmacother. 2016;84:552-558. DOI:10.1016/j.biopha.2016.09.082

[48] Moraes RC, Dias FL, Figueredo CM, Fischer RG. Association between Chronic Periodontitis and Oral/Oropharyngeal Cancer. Braz Dent J. 2016;27(3):261-266. DOI:10.1590/0103-6440201600754

[49] Javed F, Warnakulasuriya S. Is there a relationship between periodontal disease and oral cancer? A systematic review of currently available evidence. Crit Rev Oncol Hematol. 2016;97:197-205. DOI:10.1016/j.critrevonc.2015.08.018

[50] Yao QW, Zhou DS, Peng HJ, Ji P, Liu DS. Association of periodontal disease with oral cancer: a meta-analysis. Tumour Biol. 2014;35(7):7073-7077. DOI:10.1007/s13277-014-1951-8

[51] Shin YJ, Choung HW, Lee JH, Rhyu IC, Kim HD. Association of Periodontitis with Oral Cancer: A Case-Control Study. J Dent Res. 2019;98(5):526-533. doi:10.1177/0022034519827565

[52] Fitzpatrick SG, Katz J. The association between periodontal disease and cancer: a review of the literature. J Dent. 2010;38(2):83-95. DOI:10.1016/j.jdent.2009.10.007

[53] Tezal M, Sullivan MA, Reid ME, Marshall JR, Hyland A, Loree T, et al. Chronic periodontitis and the risk of tongue cancer. Arch Otolaryngol Head Neck Surg. 2007;133(5):450-454. DOI:10.1001/archotol.133.5.450

[54] Tezal M, Sullivan MA, Hyland A, Marshall JR, Stoler D, Reid ME, et al. Chronic periodontitis and the incidence of head and neck squamous cell carcinoma. Cancer Epidemiol Biomarkers Prev. 2009;18(9):2406-2412. DOI:10.1158/1055-9965.EPI-09-0334

[55] Heikkilä P, But A, Sorsa T, Haukka J. Periodontitis and cancer mortality: Register-based cohort study of 68,273 adults in 10-year follow-up. Int J Cancer. 2018;142(11):2244-2253. DOI:10.1002/ijc.31254

[56] Michaud DS, Fu Z, Shi J, Chung M. Periodontal Disease, Tooth Loss, and Cancer Risk. Epidemiol Rev. 2017;39(1):49-58. DOI:10.1093/epirev/mxx006

[57] Mager DL, Haffajee AD, Devlin PM, Norris CM, Posner MR, Goodson JM. The salivary microbiota as a diagnostic indicator of oral cancer: a descriptive, non-randomized study of cancer-free and oral squamous cell carcinoma

subjects. J Transl Med. 2005;3:27. DOI:10.1186/1479-5876-3-27

[58] Robledo-Sierra J, Ben-Amy DP, Varoni E, Bavarian R, Simonsen JL, Paster BJ, et al. World Workshop on Oral Medicine VII: Targeting the oral microbiome Part 2: Current knowledge on malignant and potentially malignant oral disorders. Oral Dis. 2019;25 Suppl 1:28-48. DOI:10.1111/odi.13107

[59] Chang C, Geng F, Shi X, Li Y, Zhang X, Zhao X, et al. The prevalence rate of periodontal pathogens and its association with oral squamous cell carcinoma. Appl Microbiol Biotechnol. 2019;103(3):1393-1404. DOI:10.1007/s00253-018-9475-6

[60] Michaud DS, Kelsey KT, Papathanasiou E, Genco CA, Giovannucci E. Periodontal disease and risk of all cancers among male never smokers: an updated analysis of the Health Professionals Follow-up Study. Ann Oncol. 2016;27(5):941-947. DOI:10.1093/annonc/mdw028

[61] Barros SP, Fahimipour F, Tarran R, Kim S, Scarel-Caminaga RM, Justice A, et al. Epigenetic reprogramming in periodontal disease: Dynamic crosstalk with potential impact in oncogenesis. Periodontol 2000. 2020;82(1):157-172. DOI:10.1111/prd.12322

[62] Mantovani A, Allavena P, Sica A, Balkwill F. Cancer-related inflammation. Nature. 2008;454:436-44. DOI: 10.1038/nature07205.

[63] Tezal M, Grossi SG, Genco RJ. Is periodontitis associated with oral neoplasms?. J Periodontol. 2005;76(3):406-410. DOI:10.1902/jop.2005.76.3.406

[64] Cekici A, Kantarci A, Hasturk H, Van Dyke TE. Inflammatory and immune pathways in the pathogenesis of periodontal disease. Periodontol 2000. 2014;64(1):57-80. DOI:10.1111/prd.12002

[65] Feller L, Altini M, Lemmer J. Inflammation in the context of oral cancer. Oral Oncol. 2013;49(9):887-892. DOI:10.1016/j.oraloncology.2013.07.003

[66] Gonda TA, Tu S, Wang TC. Chronic inflammation, the tumor microenvironment and carcinogenesis. Cell Cycle. 2009;8(13):2005-2013. DOI:10.4161/cc.8.13.8985

[67] Mascolo M, Siano M, Ilardi G, Russo D, Merolla F, De Rosa G, et al. Epigenetic disregulation in oral cancer. Int J Mol Sci. 2012;13(2):2331-2353. DOI:10.3390/ijms13022331

[68] Rodríguez-Paredes M, Esteller M. Cancer epigenetics reaches mainstream oncology. Nat Med. 2011;17(3):330-339. DOI:10.1038/nm.2305

[69] Goertzen C, Mahdi H, Laliberte C, Meirson T, Eymael D, Gil-Henn H, et al. Oral inflammation promotes oral squamous cell carcinoma invasion. Oncotarget. 2018;9(49):29047-29063. DOI:10.18632/oncotarget.25540

[70] Sahingur SE, Yeudall WA. Chemokine function in periodontal disease and oral cavity cancer. Front Immunol. 2015;6:214. DOI:10.3389/fimmu.2015.00214

[71] Karan D. Inflammasomes: Emerging Central Players in Cancer Immunology and Immunotherapy. Front Immunol. 2018;9:3028. DOI:10.3389/fimmu.2018.03028

[72] Atanasova KR, Yilmaz Ö. Prelude to oral microbes and chronic diseases: past, present and future. Microbes Infect. 2015;17(7):473-483. DOI:10.1016/j.micinf.2015.03.007

[73] Kumar J, Teoh SL, Das S, Mahakknaukrauh P. Oxidative Stress

in Oral Diseases: Understanding Its Relation with Other Systemic Diseases. Front Physiol. 2017;8:693. DOI:10.3389/fphys.2017.00693

[74] Candido J, Hagemann T. Cancer-related inflammation. J Clin Immunol. 2013;33 Suppl 1:S79-S84. DOI:10.1007/s10875-012-9847-0

[75] Repetto M, Semprine J, Boveris A, Catala A, editor. Lipid Peroxidation: Chemical Mechanism, Biological Implications and Analytical Determination. In: Lipid Peroxidation. IntechOpen; 2012. Available from: https://www.intechopen.com/books/lipid-peroxidation/lipid- peroxidation-chemical-mechanism-biological-implications-and-analytical-determination [Accessed 20-11-2020]

[76] Metgud R, Bajaj S. Altered serum and salivary C-reactive protein levels in patients with oral premalignant lesions and oral squamous cell carcinoma. Biotech Histochem. 2016;91(2):96-101. DOI:10.3109/10520295.2015.1077393

[77] Whitmore SE, Lamont RJ. Oral bacteria and cancer. PLoS Pathog. 2014;10(3):e1003933. DOI:10.1371/journal.ppat.1003933

[78] Galvão-Moreira LV, da Cruz MC. Oral microbiome, periodontitis and risk of head and neck cancer. Oral Oncol. 2016;53:17-19. DOI:10.1016/j.oraloncology.2015.11.013

[79] Katz J, Onate MD, Pauley KM, Bhattacharyya I, Cha S. Presence of Porphyromonas gingivalis in gingival squamous cell carcinoma. Int J Oral Sci. 2011;3(4):209-215. DOI:10.4248/IJOS11075

[80] Fitzsimonds ZR, Rodriguez-Hernandez CJ, Bagaitkar J, Lamont RJ. From Beyond the Pale to the Pale Riders: The Emerging Association of Bacteria with Oral Cancer. J Dent Res. 2020;99(6):604-612. DOI:10.1177/0022034520907341

Chapter 2

Periodontal Disease Associated with Genetic Disorders

Juan Wu, Wai Keung Leung and Weibin Sun

Abstract

The object of this chapter was to provide an overview including relevant research progress of some genetic disorders with periodontal manifestations. A number of genetic disorders increase patient susceptibility to periodontal disease, with the latter exhibit rather rapid and aggressive presentations. Periodontal disease, perhaps could be the first detectable sign of an undiagnosed genetic disorder. It is therefore important for dental practitioners to be familiar with genetic disorders and their impact on the periodontal tissues. This chapter reviews several genetic disorders that exhibit periodontal manifestations, including hereditary gingival fibromatosis, Papillon-Lefèvre syndrome, cyclic neutropenia, Ehlers-Danlos syndrome and hypophosphatasia.

Keywords: cyclic neutropenia, Ehlers-Danlos syndrome, genetic disorders, hereditary gingival fibromatosis, hypophosphatasia, Papillon-Lefèvre syndrome, periodontal disease

1. Introduction

Periodontal disease is an inflammatory disease that affects the gingival tissues and periodontal attachment apparatus (cementum, periodontal membrane, and alveolar bone) that surround and support the teeth [1]. In its early stage or gingivitis, the gums become swollen and red due to inflammation. In the more serious form of periodontal disease or periodontitis, which is one common chronic infection in the human mouth, loss of periodontal supportive tissue, including gingiva, periodontal ligament and alveolar bone, were evident [2] with untreated periodontitis one of the major causes of tooth loss in adults. With reference to current advances in knowledge from both biological and clinical studies since 1999 or the last International Classification of Periodontal Diseases, the 2017 World Workshop Classification system for periodontal diseases was refined and revised accordingly [3–5]. In the 2017 classification system, gingival diseases include dental biofilm-induced gingivitis and non-dental biofilm-induced gingival diseases. Periodontitis classification include necrotizing periodontal diseases, periodontitis, and periodontitis as a manifestation of systemic disease [4, 5]. The treatment of periodontal disease with systemic disease at the present date remained a significant challenge. It is paramount that correct diagnosis is made so appropriate treatment can be planned and delivered. The purpose of this chapter was to review the current literature with selected case reports concerning periodontal disease associated with genetic disorders, including hereditary gingival fibromatosis, Papillon-Lefèvre syndrome, cyclic neutropenia, Ehlers-Danlos syndrome, and hypophosphatasia. The etiology of these genetic disorders, prevalence and incidence, the clinical oral manifestations and the possible therapeutic approaches will be discussed.

2. Methodology

This chapter used a review approach aim to summarize the current literature concerning periodontal disease associated with genetic disorders, meanwhile, the chapter also provided some clinical cases including hereditary gingival fibromatosis, Papillon-Lefèvre syndrome, cyclic neutropenia, Ehlers-Danlos syndrome, and hypophosphatasia.

2.1 Literature search strategies

A review of the literature concerning periodontal disease associated with genetic disorders was conducted using PubMed, Embase, Web of Science, Google Scholar, and the Cochrane Library with no restrictions placed on country or publication date. The search involved the genetic disorders listed in the 2017 Classification System for Periodontal Diseases and Conditions [6]. The keywords used in the online searches were (the name of disorder) AND (periodontal disease OR periodontitis OR attachment loss). Additional relevant articles were also found by scanning the references of included articles as well as those citing the papers concerned.

2.2 Screening and selection criteria of studies

The identified study titles were first screened to exclude studies not relevant to periodontal disease associated with genetic disorders. For studies with apparent relevant title, the abstract would be reviewed to check and confirm potential eligibility, normally followed by careful study of the full text involved. Once eligibility is confirmed, the reference list of the included paper as well as those articles cited the latter would be reviewed for additional relevant reports. Different types of studies were included and evaluated, including case series/reports. Etiology, gene(s) involved, inheritance pattern, clinical signs and proposed therapeutic approach(es) for these periodontal diseases associated with genetic disorders were noted (**Table 1**).

In particular, five genetic disorders were given special attention: hereditary gingival fibromatosis, Papillon-Lefèvre syndrome, cyclic neutropenia, Ehlers-Danlos syndrome, and hypophosphatasia. Information regarding etiology, prevalence and incidence, clinical oral manifestations and the possible therapeutic approaches concerning these five disorders would be noted and summarized.

3. Genetic disorders that affect the periodontal tissue

According to the International Workshop in 2017, periodontal disease as a manifestation of systemic diseases is a separate disease category, systemic diseases are divided into hematological and genetic disorders [6]. Genetic disorders are caused by gene mutations or chromosome disorders that cause a change in the number or structure of chromosomes [7]. **Table 1** shows some well described genetic disorders that have a major impact on the periodontal tissue, including some disorders affecting gingival tissue (hereditary gingival fibromatosis), connective tissues (vascular Ehlers-Danlos syndrome, periodontal Ehlers-Danlos syndrome), some

Genetic disorders	IP	Gene	Etiology	Clinical oral signs/symptoms	Therapy	OMIM
Hereditary gingival fibromatosis (HGF)	AD or AR	*SOS1* *REST* *ZNF862*	Proliferative fibrous overgrowth of the gingival tissue caused by an increase in the subepithelial connective tissue elements	Proliferative fibrous overgrowth of the attached gingiva, marginal gingiva, and interdental papilla	Preventive treatment, gingivectomy, and/ or gingivoplasty	135300
Down syndrome (DS)	/	/	Trisomy chromosome 21, reduced chemotaxis and impaired phagocytosis	Gingivitis; necrotizing ulcerative gingivitis; severe periodontitis; tooth mobility	Preventive treatment and periodontal therapy	190685
Leukocyte adhesion deficiency (LAD)	AR	LAD-1: *ITGB2;* LAD-2: *SLC35C1;* LAD-3: *FERMT3*	Defects in adhesion receptors of the white blood cells and impaired phagocytosis	Severe gingival inflammation; rapidly progressive periodontitis; recurrent aphthous ulceration	Periodontal treatment +/− adjunct antibiotics, often involve extraction of primary or permanent teeth	116920 266265 607901
Papillon-Lefèvre syndrome (PLS)	AR	*CTSC*	Mutated cathepsin-c gene, impaired neutrophil function	Aggressive periodontal breakdown; premature loss of teeth	Periodontal treatment with adjunct antibiotics; according to the age of onset, may involve extraction of deciduous teeth 6 months prior to eruption of permanent successors	245000
Haim-Munk syndrome (HMS)	AR	*CTSC*	Mutation of gene encoding for cathepsin-c, impaired neutrophil function	Severe gingival inflammation; periodontitis; early loss of teeth	Extraction of the primary teeth combined with adjunct antibiotics and periodontal therapy	245010
Chediak-Higashi syndrome (CHS)	AR	*LYST*	Impaired lysis of phagocytized bacteria, resulting in recurrent bacterial respiratory and other infections and oculocutaneous albinism.	Severe gingivitis; early-onset periodontitis; oral ulcerations	The disease posts great challenges to periodontal management: intensive prevention, meticulous mechanical therapy with antibiotics and chemical plaque control	214500
Severe congenital neutronpenia (SCN),	AR or AD	*ELANE* and *HAX1*	An arrest in myeloid maturation at the promyelocyte	Gingival inflammation; severe alveolar bone loss; early loss of	Conventional periodontal treatment with antibiotics	610738

Genetic disorders	IP	Gene	Etiology	Clinical oral signs/symptoms	Therapy	OMIM
Kostmann syndrome			stage in the bone marrow	teeth; oral ulcerations		
Cyclic neutron-penia (CN)	AD	*ELANE*	Cyclical decrease in the number of circulating neutrophils	Gingival inflammation; severe periodontitis; oral ulcers	Periodontal therapy followed by monthly debridement and extra therapy during neutropenic episodes; chlorhexidine rinsing	162800
Cohen syndrome	AR	*VPS13B*	Abnormal protein glycosylation and Golgi dysfunction	Periodontal disease	Prevention and conventional periodontal therapy	216550
Ehlers-Danlos syndrome (Vascular type, vEDS)	AD	*COL3A1* or *COL1A1*	Defective collagen synthesis	Gingival recession; gingival fragility	Periodontal therapy followed by mechanical and chemical plaque control	130050
Ehlers-Danlos syndrome (Periodontal type, pEDS)	AD	*C1R* or *C1S*	Secretion or release of active C1r serine protease in the extracellular space	Severe and intractable periodontitis of early onset; lack of attached gingiva	Periodontal therapy with strict biofilm management to stop the plaque-associated periodontal hyperinflammation and probably the subsequent bone and tooth loss	130080
Glycogen storage disease 1b (GSD 1b)	AR	*SLC37A4*	Deficiency of glucose-6-phosphate translocase	Oral ulcers; hyperplastic gingiva; periodontal infections; prolonged bleeding	Preventive treatment, periodontal therapy and control of gingival disease	232220
Hypophos-phatasia (HPP)	AD or AR	*ALPL*	Decreased activity of tissue nonspecific alkaline phosphatase	Absence of root cementum; premature exfoliation of deciduous teeth	Periodontal therapy with possible extraction of involved primary teeth and more conservative treatment on permanent teeth	146300

AD, autosomal dominant; ALPL, *alkaline phosphatase, biomineralization associated gene; AR, autosomal recessive;* C1R, *complement 1 subunit r gene;* C1S, *complement 1 subunit s gene;* COL1A1, *collagen type I alpha 1 chain gene;* COL3A1, collagen type III alpha 1 chain gene; CTSC, *cathepsin C gene; ELANE, elastase, neutrophil expressed gene; FERMT3, fermitin family member 3 gene; HAX1, HCLS1-associated protein X-1 gene; HCLS1, hematopoietic cell-specific lyn substrate 1; IP, inheritance pattern; ITGB2, integrin subunit beta 2 gene; LYST, lysosomal trafficking regulator gene; OMIM,* online Mendelian Inheritance in man; *RE1, transcriptional repressor element-1,* REST, *RE1-silencing transcription factor gene;* SLC35C1, *solute carrier family 35 member C1 gene;* SLC37A4, *solute carrier family 37 member 4 gene;* SOS, *son of sevenless genes;* SOS1, SOS *Ras/Rac guanine nucleotide exchange factor 1 gene;* VPS13B, *vacuolar protein sorting 13 homolog B gene;* ZNF862, *Zinc finger protein 862 gene.*

Table 1.
Periodontal disease associated with genetic disorders.

diseases associated with immunologic disorders (Down syndrome, leukocyte adhesion deficiency, Papillon-Lefèvre syndrome, Haim-Munk syndrome, Chediak-Higashi syndrome, Severe congenital neutropenia, cyclic neutropenia, Cohen syndrome) and metabolic disorders (glycogen storage disease 1b, hypophosphatasia) [6, 8–12].

3.1 Hereditary gingival fibromatosis

Hereditary gingival fibromatosis (HGF) is a rare, hereditary disorder characterized by a benign, non-hemorrhagic, localized or generalized fibrous enlargement of free and attached gingivae with slow progression, and was initially reported by Goddard and Gross in 1856 [13, 14]. It has been designated by such terms as gingivostomatosis, elephantiasis, idiopathic fibromatosis, hereditary gingival hyperplasia, idiopathic gingival enlargement, and congenital familial fibromatosis. The prevalence is unknown, the incidence is 1:175,000 according to phenotype and 1:350,000 according to genotype, and equal between males and females. HGF is commonly described as an isolated disorder (non-syndromic), or it can develop as a part of a syndrome (syndromic) like Cowden's syndrome, Zimmermann-laband syndrome, Cross syndrome, Rutherford syndrome, Ramon syndrome, Jones syndrome, Costello syndrome, Ectro-amelia syndrome, and hyaline fibromatosis syndrome [15]. In this part, we mainly discuss non-syndromic HGF.

3.1.1 Etiology and pathogenesis

The mode of HGF inheritance is still controversial, while it is generally considered to be an autosomal dominant disease, there are a few studies demonstrating that it may also follow an autosomal recessive pattern [16]. **Figure 1** shows a Chinese pedigree with non-syndromic HGF in an autosomal dominant mode. As reported earlier, four loci (2p22.1 [MIM: 135300], 2p23.3-p22.3 [MIM: 609955], 5q13-q22 [MIM: 605544] and 11p15 [MIM: 611010]) were recognized to be related with HGF [17–20], while SOS Ras/Rac guanine nucleotide exchange factor 1 gene (*SOS1*) (MIM: 182530) heterozygous frameshift mutation was acknowledged causing autosomal dominant HGF in a Brazilian family [21]. From three independent families, two Turkish and one American, protein truncating mutations of RE1-silencing transcription factor or *REST* gene (MIM: 600571) were identified to cause autosomal dominant HGF [22]. In our department, we identified seventeen autosomal dominant non-syndromic HGF patients from a Chinese family (**Figure 1**). Across three generations, whole-exome sequencing then genetic co-segregation analysis were performed identifying an original Zinc finger protein 862 (*ZNF862*) gene heterozygous missense mutation to be the cause of the genetic problem [23].

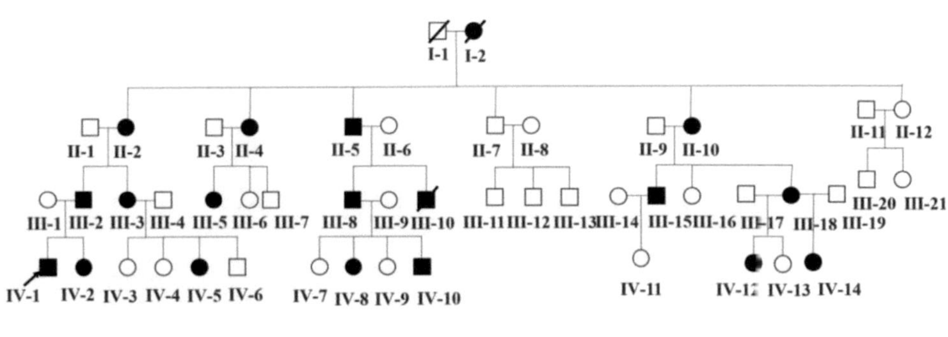

Figure 1.
A Chinese pedigree with non-syndromic hereditary gingival fibromatosis (HGF).

The pathophysiologic mechanisms underpinning HGF remain elusive. Nonetheless, extracellular matrix overproduction involving major component of collagen type I was believed to be a cause of the gingival fibroblast overgrowth phenotype; on the other hand, increased production of TIMP-1 appeared to be associated with excessive collagen I accumulation in HGF fibroblasts [24, 25]. Also, Martelli-Junior and coworkers claimed that TGF-β1, IL-6 and perhaps other specific growth factors overproduction in fibroblasts might play pivotal roles in unwarranted collagen I synthesis [26].

3.1.2 Clinical manifestations

The onset of the gingival overgrowth usually coincides with the eruption of permanent incisors, while under rare circumstances, HGF can present at birth (**Figures 2–4**). The overgrowth affects the attached gingiva as well as the gingival margin and the interdental papillae. The facial and lingual surfaces of the permanent teeth are generally affected, the enlarged gingiva is usually firm, smooth and occasionally nodular, with minimal or no inflammation and normal or pale in color. The upper gingiva is more severely affected and may prevent the eruption of the teeth. In severe cases, the teeth are almost completely covered. The firm yet painless enlargement of the gingiva does not commonly affect the alveolar bone but can lead

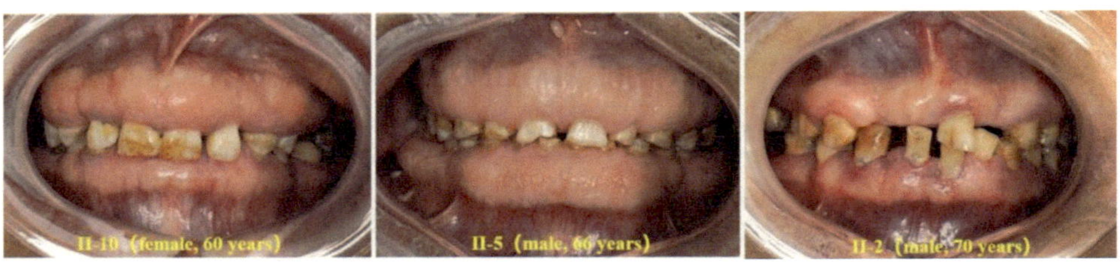

Figure 2.
HGF in Chinese elderlies.

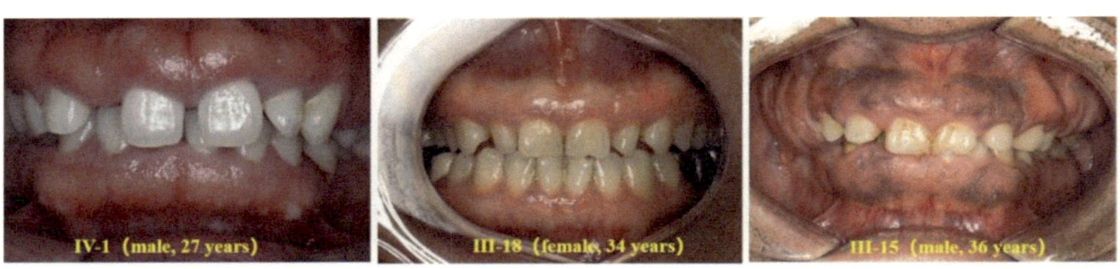

Figure 3.
HGF in Chinese adults.

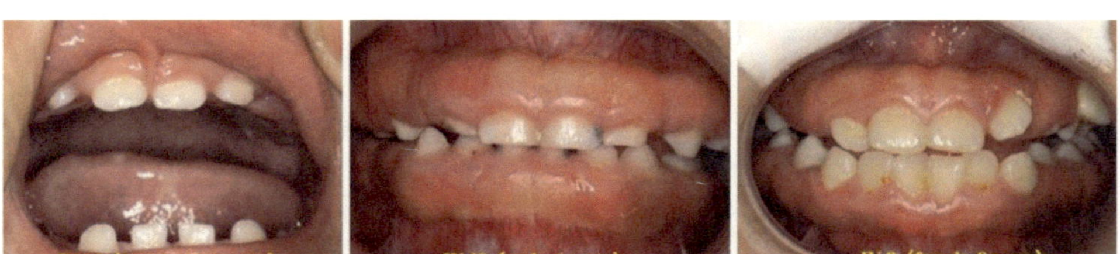

Figure 4.
HGF in Chinese children.

to the development of pseudo-pockets, which facilitate plaque accumulation due to suboptimal daily oral hygiene [13–16].

Enlarged gingival tissues due to HGF cause functional and esthetic problems. The lesion partially and at times totally cover the crowns of teeth causing pseudo-pocketing. In extreme situations, HGF could delay or even impede tooth eruption, causing diastemas, mal-position/−alignment of teeth, cross−/open-bite, excessive lip support including vermillion eversion, and/or incompetence lips. Common clinical complications secondary to gingival enlargement including but not limited to difficulties in speech, mastication, and occlusion, as well as changes in facial features. Interestingly, the condition may disappear or regress with the loss of teeth, thus suggesting that the presence of teeth might serve as one condition for the development of HGF [13–16].

3.1.3 Diagnosis

Diagnosis of HGF is usually based on clinical findings, a generalized severe gingival overgrowth without medication history, and the familial aggregation of HGF can assist in early diagnosis [27, 28]. The differential diagnosis should include gingival hyperplasia due to phenytoin, nifedipine and cyclosporine and gingival fibromatosis, which may occur as part of other genetic syndromes.

HGF related gingival fibrous enlargement typically display marked increase in submucosal connective tissue histologically. The involved connective tissue looks densely collagenized, populated scantly with fibroblasts, avascular and with signs indicating minimal inflammatory infiltrate. The overlying dense epithelial layer appears hyperkeratotic with elongated rete pegs. In situation when abnormal thickening of the stratum spinosum or prickle cell layer, i.e. acanthosis of the HGF involved epithelium, areas with chronic inflammation within the epithelium can sometimes be detected [27, 29].

3.1.4 Treatment

The maintenance of good oral hygiene and plaque control is fundamental. Treatments vary according to the degree of severity of gingival enlargement and different types of treatment modality could be employed for the excision, including conventional surgery, electrosurgery, apically positioned flap and laser ablation [14, 27, 30].

For HGF patients with mild gingival hyperplasia, supportive periodontal therapy is recommended every 3 months.

For HGF patients with modern-severe gingival hyperplasia, periodontal surgery is required (**Figures 5** and **6**), including gingivectomy, gingivoplasty, and flap surgery. Some literature indicated that laser can also be used to remove hyperplastic gingival, with higher patient comfort and less trauma. Recurrence after surgical treatment was observed within 3–10 years, and children and adolescents are more likely to recurrence than adults. Therefore, regular follow-up and good oral hygiene are very important.

For HGF patients with severe gingival hyperplasia deformation, surgical interventions that may be required include tooth extraction, osteoplasty and ostectomy.

A comprehensive medical and family history, along with clinical examination can aid early HGF diagnosis because the latter often associates with a few extra-oral features on top of familial aggregation. Gingivectomy is often the treatment of choice while long-term follow-up post-surgery is recommended for the relatively high probability of HGF recurrence.

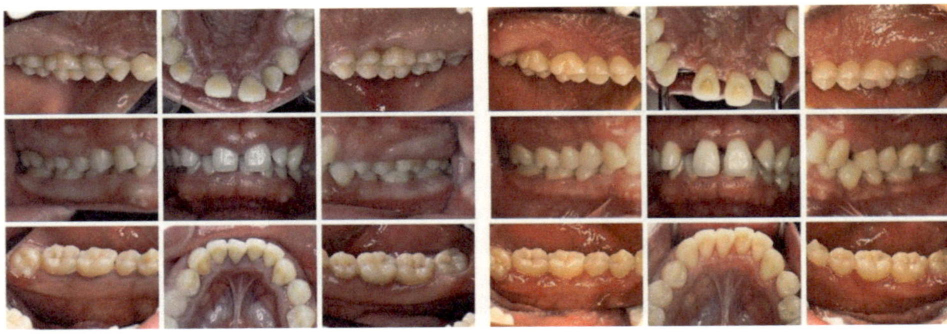

Figure 5.
Periodontal surgery (gingivectomy, gingivoplasty, and flap surgery) in a Chinese HGF patient (IV-1, ***Figures 1*** *and 3; pre-operation [left panels: Set of nine intra-oral photographs] and 6 months follow-up [right hand panels]).*

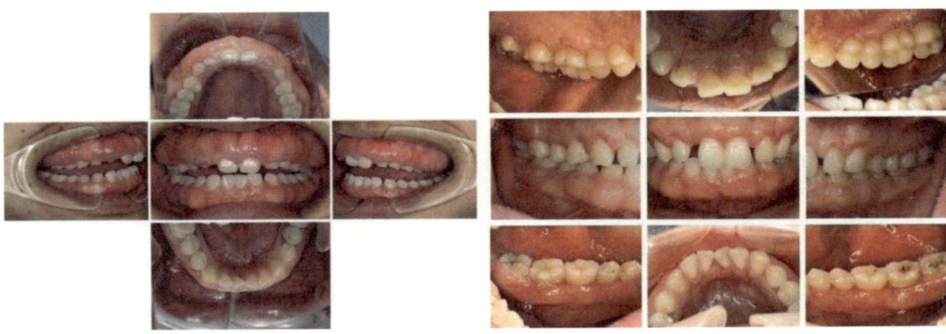

Figure 6.
Periodontal surgery (gingivectomy, gingivoplasty, and flap surgery) in a Chinese HGF patient (IV-2, ***Figure 1****; pre-operation [right hand panels] and 2 years follow-up [left hand panels]).*

3.2 Papillon-Lefèvre syndrome

Papillon-Lefèvre syndrome (PLS), first reported in a French family by physicians Papillon and Lefèvre in 1924, is an autosomal recessive disorder characterized by diffuse palmoplantar erythematous, fissured hyperkeratosis, and aggressive periodontal disease that starts in the early periods of childhood. It has been designated by such terms as "keratoris palmoplantaris" and "hyperkeratosis palmoplantaris" [31, 32]. Periodontitis occurs with the early loss of deciduous teeth at the age of 2 to 4 years, followed by the loss of permanent teeth during adolescence. The prevalence is unknown, more than 300 families worldwide have been reported in the medical literature [33]. In the general population, PLS occurs in approximately one to four individuals per million, and consanguinity is reported as a significant risk factor and has been demonstrated in 20–40% of PLS patients [34]. With reference to 124 PLS cases, Haneke raise the following generalizations: (1) females and males appeared equally affected; (2) no racial predominance of the condition, apparently, could be observable; (3) however, consanguinity was associated with a third of the cases; and (4) other than periodontitis, increased susceptibility to other infections was observed in a quarter of PLS patients [32].

3.2.1 Etiology and pathogenesis

PLS is caused by changes (alterations) in *CTSC* gene, which encodes cathepsin C, a lysosomal protease capable of removing dipeptides from the amino-terminus portion of its respective substrates [35]. The protein is expressed at high levels in various immune cells and certain bodily areas affected by PLS, including epithelial cells, that form the protective outer layer of the skin (epidermis), such as of the palms, soles, and knees, as well as certain cells of the gingiva. To date, more than 90 mutations in *CTSC* have been reported associate with PLS with the majority being located between Exons 5 and 7, the region encoding the heavy chain domain of cathepsin C that controls its enzymatic activity. Cathepsin C activity is proposed to play a key role in the epithelial differentiation and desquamation, while the inappropriate genetic alterations may result in nearly complete loss of cathepsin C enzymatic activity in homozygous individuals with the disease, or correspondently reduced activity of the enzyme in the family members who are heterozygous carriers [36, 37]. The present research group reported a PLS patient with a 110 kb deletion (Chr11: 88032292:88142997 [NC_000011]) and a nonsense mutation exists (Gln182Ter, CAG > TAG) in the fourth exon of the *CTSC* gene [38].

Another important related periodontitis etiologic factor is an alteration of the host defense owing to decreased function of lymphocytes, polymorphonuclear leucocytes or monocytes. However, research into such factors has not led to consistent findings and more research is necessary to decipher the underlying mechanisms that lead to the development of clinical manifestation observed in PLS [39, 40]. The subgingival plaque sampled from periodontal pockets of PLS patients resembled typical periodontitis-associated microflora, i.e. predominant gram-negative anaerobic microbes, including *Porphyromonas gingivalis* and spirochetes. Recent microbiologic report indicated that *Aggregatibacter actinomycetemcomitans* was detectable in periodontal sites in PLS patients [41].

3.2.2 Clinical manifestations

Patients with PLS present first clinical signs in the oral cavity as soon as the deciduous teeth erupt [34, 36]. Oral manifestations become apparent by the age of 2 to 3 years with rapid periodontal destruction: plaque accumulation, obvious gingival inflammation and bleeding, periodontal abscess, deep periodontal pocket formation, alveolar bone resorption, loose teeth, halitosis, following by premature exfoliation of all deciduous teeth by the age of 4 to 5 years (**Figure 7**) [38]. Radiographic investigations show generalized alveolar bone loss and migration of teeth whit no evidence of root resorption (**Figure 8**). Inflammation disappears during the edentulous period, but the disease process reappears when permanent dentition erupts, with the affected losing most of the teeth at teenage (**Figure 9**).

PLS is characterized by development of hyperkeratosis or dry scaly skin patches at early age of one to five years old. These patches usually confined to palms and

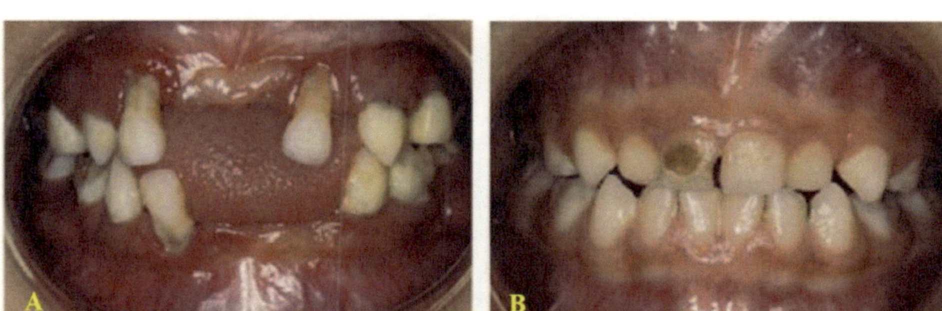

Figure 7.
Oral manifestations of a Papillon-Lefèvre syndrome (PLS) patient (3 years) with serious periodontitis (A) and her fraternal twin sister with healthy periodontal tissue (B).

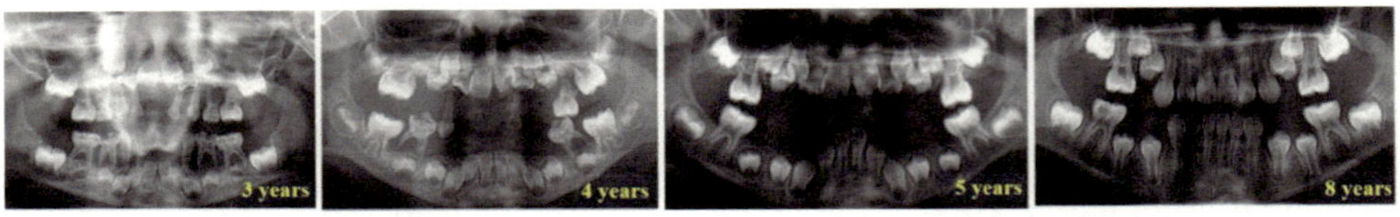

Figure 8.
*Panoramic radiographs of the PLS patient in **Figure 7** when she was 3–5, or 8 years old.*

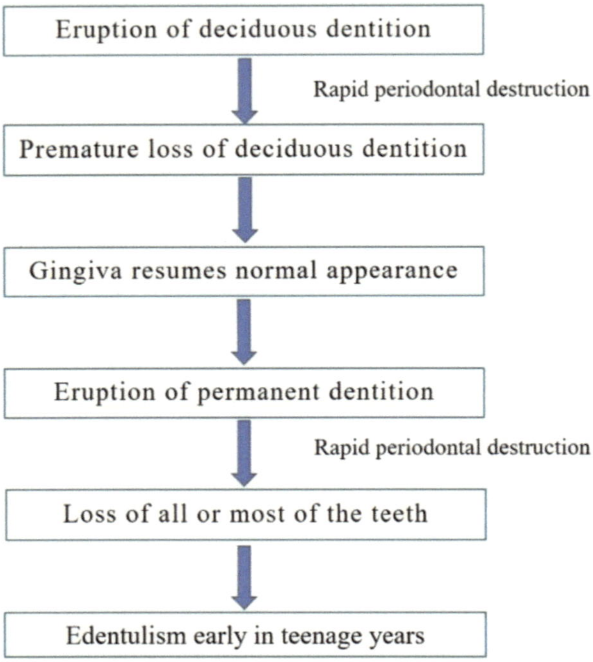

Figure 9.
Flow chart of oral manifestations of PLS.

soles, but may spread to knees and elbows. In rare occasions, upper portions of hands and feet, eyelids, lips, cheeks, and/or other bodily surfaces may also be affected. Affected skin may appear unusually thick and red, but variation in texture and color is possible. Skin lesions may worsen upon exposure to cold which lead to pain upon movement like walking. Other symptoms that may accompany the condition are hyperhidrosis, nail dystrophy, cranial calcification, and increased susceptibility to infections. Most patients show susceptibility to mild skin infections like pyodermas or furunculosis. Severe infections like pyogenic liver abscess or pneumonia, and malignancies like melanoma have been reported in PLS patients [34, 42, 43].

3.2.3 Diagnosis

Early diagnosis and prompt treatment can potentially prevent aggressive periodontitis, tooth loss, and improve overall quality of life of patients with PLS [34, 36, 44]. PLS becomes clinically apparent at 1–5 years old; palmar-plantar hyperkeratosis or dry scaly patches of palms and soles, together with severe, aggressive, or rapidly progressing periodontitis are considered its main clinical features, with or without additional symptoms like pyogenic skin infections, nail dystrophies, and hyperhidrosis. Radiographic examination of advanced PLS cases reveal severe loss of the alveolar bone, and teeth appear to be "floating in air" (**Figure 8**).

Differential diagnoses should include Haim-Munk syndrome, Chediak-Higashi syndrome, juvenile periodontitis, and so on (**Table 1**). Haim-Munk syndrome (HMS) is a skin condition caused by *CTSC* mutation. It is an extremely rare disorder of keratinization of recessive inheritance that manifests with scaly, red, and thickened patches of the skin of soles of the feet and palms of the hands, pes planus, arachnodactyly, acroosteolysis, atrophic changes of nails, a radiographic deformity of fingers, recurrent abscess formations, and a severe 'early-onset' periodontitis [45].

Neutrophil function tests reveal anomalies of chemotaxis and phagocytosis by polymorphonuclear leukocytes. Skin biopsy shows hyperkeratosis with focal parakeratosis, moderate perivascular infiltration, hypergranulosis, and acanthosis. Biochemical analysis reveals a loss of *CTSC* activity. Molecular genetic testing can confirm a diagnosis. Molecular genetic testing can detect alterations in the *CTSC* gene known to cause PLS, but is available only as a diagnostic service at specialized laboratories [36, 44].

3.2.4 Treatment

A multidisciplinary approach involving the dermatologist, pediatrician, pediatric dentist, periodontist, and prosthodontist is important for the overall care of patient with PLS [34, 46]. Genetic counseling may be of benefit for affected individuals and their families. Psychosocial support is recommended for the entire family as well. Oral retinoids with aims to attenuate palmoplantar keratoderma and to diminish alveolar bone lysis remained the main line of the therapy. Oral hygiene, chemical plaque control with or without antibiotics are the recommended therapeutic protocol for reducing periodontitis progression. Eventually, primary or terminally periodontal involved teeth are extracted. Antibiotic therapy is also used in the treatment of recurrent infections. Etretinate (a synthetic retinoid) shows promising results in the treatment of PLS.

Successful periodontal management of PLS patients is the key to improve the prognosis of the dentition, preventing or delaying primary and permanent tooth loss. During the past decades, dental treatment efforts other than extraction have been attempted in PLS patients. Several articles have been published on the treatment of PLS. Ullbro et al. proposed a mode of periodontal therapy of patients with PLS [47] (**Table 2**).

Deciduous dentition	Permanent dentition
Three-monthly oral hygiene instructions and prophylaxis	Three-monthly oral hygiene instructions and prophylaxis
To extract teeth with advanced periodontal involvement	Twice daily rinsing with chlorhexidine gluconate 0.2% mouthwash
All primary teeth to be extracted at least 6 months prior to eruption of the permanent successor; with 2 weeks antibiotic regimen post extraction: amoxicillin + clavulanic acid, 20–40 mg/kg/d, q8H	Teeth with moderate periodontitis (bone loss <30% root length, probing pocket depths <5 mm): antibiotic adjunct non-surgical periodontal therapy, i.e. amoxicillin (20–50 mg/kg/d) + metronidazole (15–35 mg/kg/d), q8H × 4 weeks; followed by monthly prophylaxis
	Teeth with advanced periodontitis (bone less >30% root length, probing pocket depth > 6 mm): consider extraction

Table 2.
Suggested mode of periodontal therapy for patients with Papillon-Lefèvre syndrome (PLS). Adopted from Ullbro et al. [47].

Most PLS patients ended up edentulous at an early age and were presented with rehabilitation problems due to severely atrophic thin alveolar ridges. Various pre-prosthetic surgical management approaches are introduced to maximize retention and stability of dentures. Along such line, dental implants are also advocated for enhancing stability and retention of prosthesis, improving comfort, masticatory efficiency and perhaps esthetics. Reports concerning installation of titanium implants in PLS patients with treated severe periodontitis to support and retain oral reconstructions indicated under good care and dedications in prevention or oral health maintenance, indicated the approach could be successful [48, 49].

3.2.5 Genetic counseling

Transmission is autosomal recessive. Genetic counseling should be offered to the parents of an affected individual informing them that 25% of their future offspring could inherit the disease-causing mutation.

3.2.6 Prognosis

Despite meticulous dental care, PLS patients eventually become edentulous at the beginning of adulthood while their life expectancy is normal [32, 42, 46].

3.3 Cyclic neutropenia

Neutropenia (absolute neutrophil count or ANC $<1.5 \times 10^9/L$), includes diagnoses ranging from normal variants like benign ethnic neutropenia to life-threatening acquired or congenital disorders like agranulocytosis. The biological consequences depend mainly on neutropenia severity and corresponding responses from the affected individual: e.g. an ANC of $1.0–1.5 \times 10^9/L$ does not normally impair host defense so far enough normally functioning neutrophils could be produced by bone marrow when needed, however the underlying cause of the low ANC need to be investigated; an ANC of $0.5–1.0 \times 10^9/L$ may increase infections risk but only if other immune defense element of the affected individual are also impaired; while an ANC of $0.2–0.5 \times 10^9/L$ normally associates with increased infections risk in most patients, an ANC $\leq 0.2 \times 10^9/L$, i.e. agranulocytosis, often implies susceptibility to opportunistic infection with high risk of severe, life threatening consequences [50].

Cyclic neutropenia (CN), first described in 1910 based on the recurrence of neutropenia, fever, and mouth ulcers in a 19-month-old boy, is a rare hematologic disease characterized by regular oscillations in blood neutrophil counts from normal levels (ANC $> 1.5 \times 10^9/L$) to severe neutropenia (ANC $< 0.2 \times 10^9/L$), usually with a cycle length of about 21 days, and lasts for 3–6 days at a time [51]. It has been designated by such terms as "cyclic hematopoiesis", "human cyclic neutropenia", and "periodic neutropenia". During intervals of neutropenia, affected patients exhibit fever, mouth ulcers and are at risk for opportunistic infection. CN affects males and females in equal numbers, and the prevalence is unknown. Most cases of CN are thought to be present at birth (congenital); however, in some cases, the diagnosis may not become obvious until childhood, adolescence, or early adulthood [52, 53].

3.3.1 Etiology and pathogenesis

As mentioned above, CN may be congenital or acquired. Congenital cases include sporadic CN without apparent causes [54, 55], inherited cases transmitted in an autosomal dominant trait related to mutations in the elastase, neutrophil expressed or gene encoding neutrophil elastase. Heterozygous mutations in *ELANE* gene have been reported in a high frequency of single base pair/amino acid mutations and identified in 80–100% of patients with CN. Neutrophil elastase is synthesized and packaged in promyelocytes at an early stage in neutrophil development. Mutations in the *ELANE* gene induce unfolded protein response-associated apoptosis at the promyelocyte stage and result in ineffective myelopoiesis, and bone marrow fail to maintain consistent production of mature neutrophils. Severe neutropenia recurs when the bone marrow supply is exhausted [56, 57].

3.3.2 Clinical manifestations

The signs and symptoms of CN usually appear at birth or shortly after, and the major clinical problem associated with neutropenia is recurrence of bacterial infections. Opportunistic infections can occur during ANC reduction, with the main clinical manifestations of fever, malaise, headache, anorexia, pharyngitis, tonsillitis, skin infections (**Figure 10**), and swollen lymph nodes, sepsis, ulcers of the oral mucous membrane (**Figure 11**), periodontal inflammation and severe periodontitis (**Figure 12**). when ANC <500/μL for more than 7 days within the cycle, patients regularly have painful mouth ulcers, upper respiratory tract infections, skin abscesses, and suffer from malaise, whereas severe infections are very rare. Oral manifestations usually occur around early childhood, systemic symptoms, such as fever, generally diminish after adolescence, but adults with CN continue to experience oral ulcers, gingivitis, and periodontitis [52, 58].

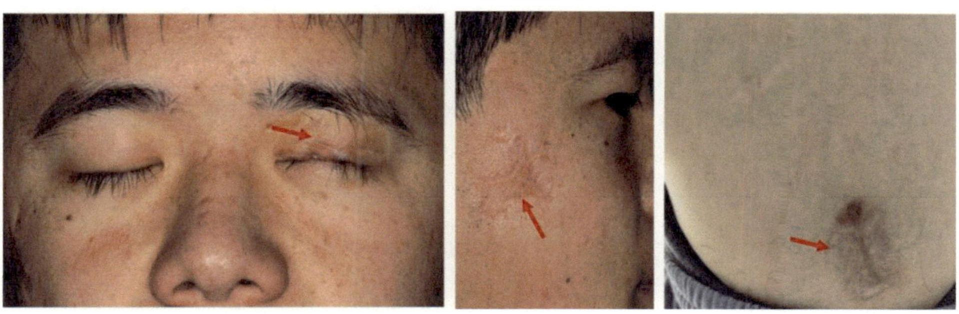

Figure 10.
Scar formation after slow healing skin infections with a Chinese male (25 years old) with cyclic neutropenia (CN).

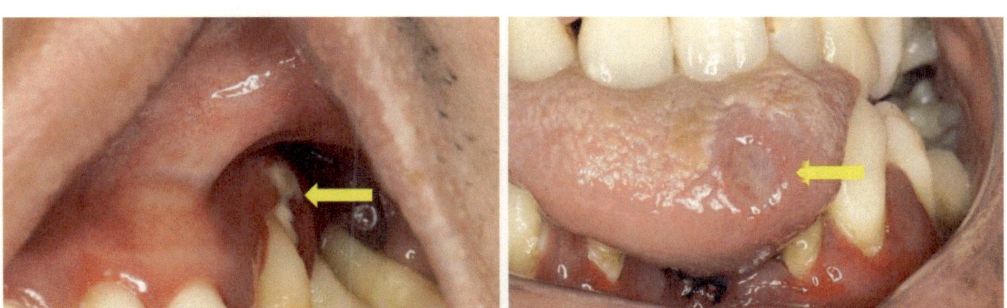

Figure 11.
*Oral ulcers in the Chinese male (**Figure 10**) with CN.*

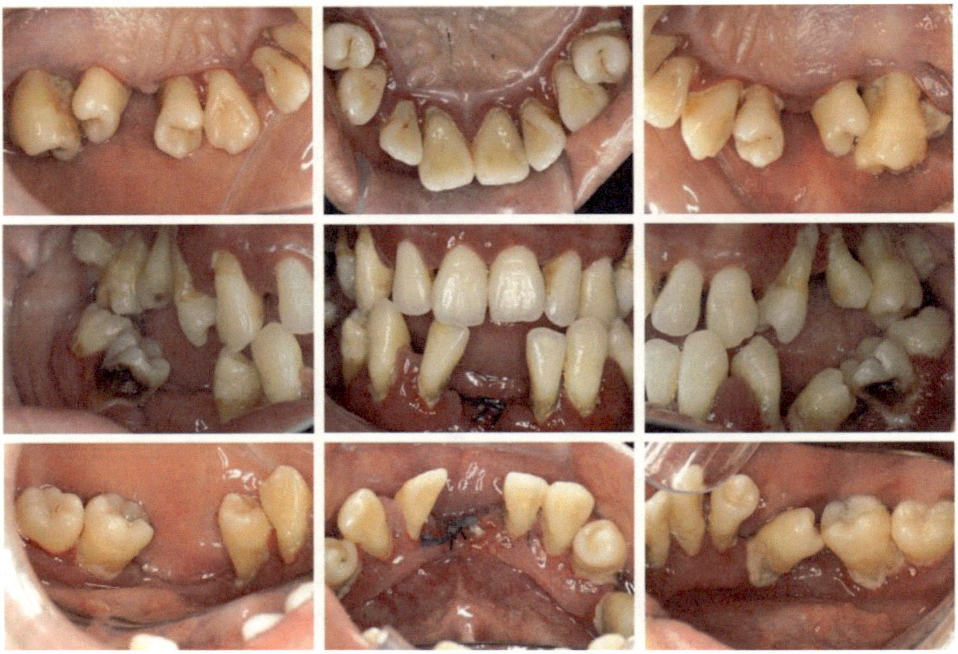

Figure 12.
*Oral manifestations of the CN patient (**Figure 10**) with serious periodontitis.*

3.3.3 Diagnosis

CN diagnosis is often made based upon detailed history taking followed by careful clinical examination and thorough evaluation of all information collected. Then the diagnosis may be confirmed by 2–3 times/week neutrophil count monitoring over six weeks. Individuals with CN should preferably be genetically confirmed by assaying corresponding mutations in the *ELANE* gene [50, 59].

Typical CN diagnostic flow includes:

1. Medical history and physical examination: recurrent infections, oral ulcers, periodontal inflammation;

2. Complete blood cells count: circulating neutrophils vary between zero to almost normal count. ANC < 500 cells/μL and occurs every 21 days, lasting 3 to 6 days at a time. Monocytes, platelets, lymphocytes and reticulocytes also cycle with the same frequency. Monitoring of ANC 2 to 3 times per week for 6 weeks (**Figure 13**);

3. Family history aid to evaluate patients with CN;

4. Genetic testing for mutations in *ELANE*.

3.3.4 Treatment

Prompt, appropriate treatment of the infections associated with CN is important, including symptomatic and supportive treatment. Careful oral and dental care is also required. In addition, individuals with CN should avoid activities that may cause minor injuries [50, 59].

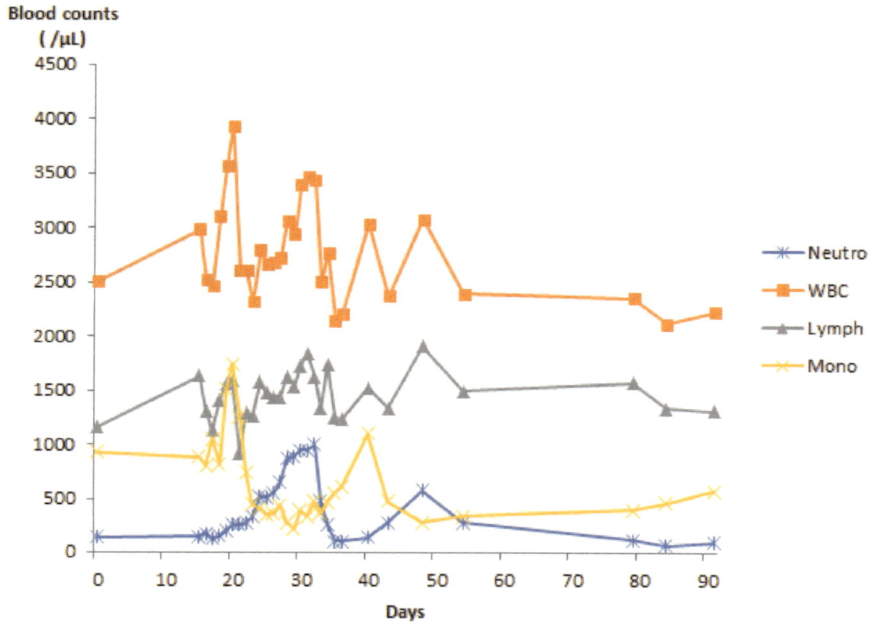

Figure 13.
*Diagnostic monitoring the changes in white blood cells (WBC), neutrophils, lymphocytes, and monocytes over a course of three months concerning the CN patient (**Figure 10**).*

Treatment with granulocyte colony-stimulating factor (G-CSF), also called Neupogen, is effective in raising blood neutrophil counts in CN patients. G-CSF treatment with G-CSF in patients with CN does not abrogate cycling, but increases the ANC, shortens the cycle periodicity from the usual 21 days to about 14 days, and prevents serious infections, reduces the symptoms and problems of infections in almost all patients [60].

Professional removal of dental plaque and calculus should be recommended monthly and during the neutropenic episodes, antibiotics may be given in order to prevent oral infection.

3.3.5 Genetic counseling

Genetic counseling is recommended for individuals with inherited forms of CN and their families, in particular the fact regarding 50% chance for CN offsprings from affected individual need to be discussed.

3.3.6 Prognosis

The development of CN is usually benign compared to autoimmune, congenital or idiopathic neutropenia. CN systemic symptoms e.g. recurrent fevers often diminish post adolescence but CN adults remained prone to oral ulcers, gingivitis, periodontitis, and various oral/facial infections [50–52].

3.4 Periodontal Ehlers-Danlos syndrome

Ehlers–Danlos syndromes (EDS) are clinically and genetically heterogeneous rare hereditary disorders categorized by varying degrees of connective tissue fragility, principally affecting skin, ligaments, blood vessels, and internal organs [61, 62]. Main clinical features comprise tissue fragility, skin extensibility, and joint hypermobility.

EDS was named by dermatologists Edvard Ehlers in 1901 and Henri-Alexandre Danlos in 1908. In 2017, the international EDS consortium published a revised EDS classification system with specific emphasis on molecular diagnosis as well as identification of causative genetic variants. The new classification recognizes 13 subtypes and periodontal manifestations are commonly observed in patients with periodontal Ehlers-Danlos syndrome (pEDS), also known as EDS type VIII, Ehlers-Danlos Syndrome, Periodontitis Type or Ehlers-Danlos Syndrome Periodontal Type [63, 64].

pEDS was considered a distinct EDS subtype [65] characterized by severe periodontitis with early disease onset with premature tooth loss, extra-orally includes pretibial hyperpigmented scarring, easy bruising and joint hypermobility. pEDS is an extremely rare EDS subtype with autosomal dominant inheritance. pEDS affects males and females in equal numbers, and the prevalence is unknown, more than 100 pEDS patients were reported [63, 64, 66].

3.4.1 Etiology and pathogenesis

pEDS was be caused by heterozygous mutations in complement 1 subunit genes *C1R* and *C1S* [67], and our understanding of the pathophysiological mechanisms underlying these conditions remains very limited. Experimental evidence suggests that it is linked to secretion or release of active C1r serine protease in the extracellular space. This mechanism may cause gingival hyperinflammation in response to mild biofilm accumulation, and subsequently rapidly progressing periodontal destruction [68].

3.4.2 Clinical manifestations

A systematic review was conducted in 2017 about the clinical manifestations of pEDS, and **Table 3** shows the clinical features in 93 pEDS patients with *C1R*/*C1S* mutation [64, 66].

Features	Prevalence (%)
Oral	
Early severe periodontitis	99
Gingival recession	98
Lack of attached gingiva	93
Skin	
Easy bruising	95
Pretibial discoloration	80
(Mild)skin fragility	80
Prominent vasculature	50
Abnormal scarring	50
Joint	
Joint hypermobility	44
Joint pain	31
Flat feet	30
Scoliosis	22

Table 3.
Clinical features of periodontal Ehlers-Danlos syndrome (pEDS).

Typical clinical features of pEDS are:

1. Oral features: i) early severe periodontitis (**Figure 14**) - the age of first tooth loss was between 2 and 30 years; the age of complete tooth loss was between 14 and 48 years (**Figure 15**); and 16% patients with pEDS (age < 10 years) have prepubertal periodontitis; ii) gingival recession with visible dental root, due to gingival thinning with or without destruction of the underlying periodontal bone; iii) lack of attached gingiva.

2. Skin features: i) easy bruising; ii) pretibial discoloration with nonspecific dermal consistent with trauma and hemosiderin deposition (**Figure 16**); iii) skin fragility; iv) prominent vasculature; v) abnormal scarring (**Figure 16**).

3. Joint features: i) joint hypermobility; ii) joint pain; iii) flat feet; iv) scoliosis.

4. Other features including recurrent infection, hernia, aneurysms, autoimmune disorder, organ rupture and leukoencephalopathy.

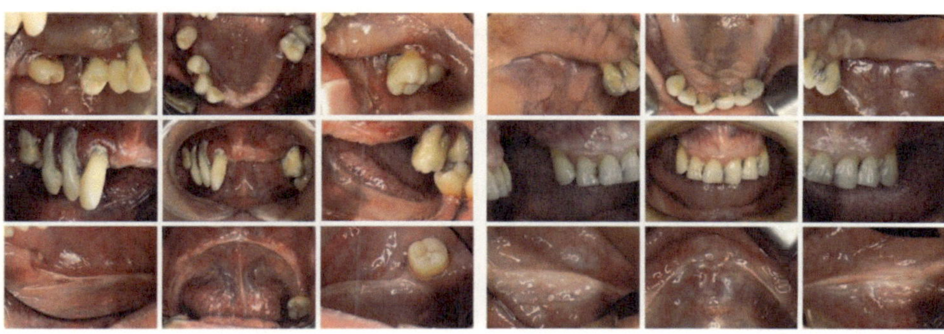

Figure 14.
Oral manifestations of periodontal Ehlers-Danlos syndrome (pEDS) patients with serious periodontitis. Left panels (set of nine intra-oral photographs) were from a Chinese male, 24 years with pEDS; right panels were from of his mother who also suffered from pEDS [69].

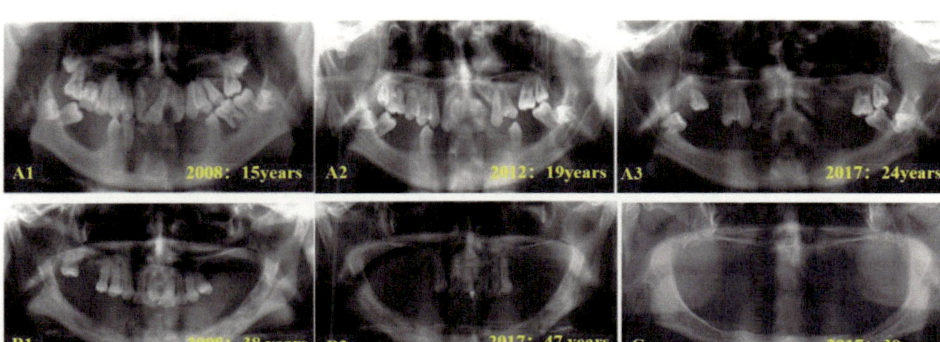

Figure 15.
*Orthopantomographs (OPG) of pEDS patients with severe alveolar bone loss, atrophic edentulous ridges. A1, A2, A3 were OPG images from the Chinese male (**Figure 14**, left panels) with pEDS in 2008, 2012 or 2017. B1 and B2 were OPG images of his mother with pEDS (**Figure 14**, right panels) in 2008 or 2017. C was OPG image from the affected maternal uncle who also has pEDS in 2017 [69].*

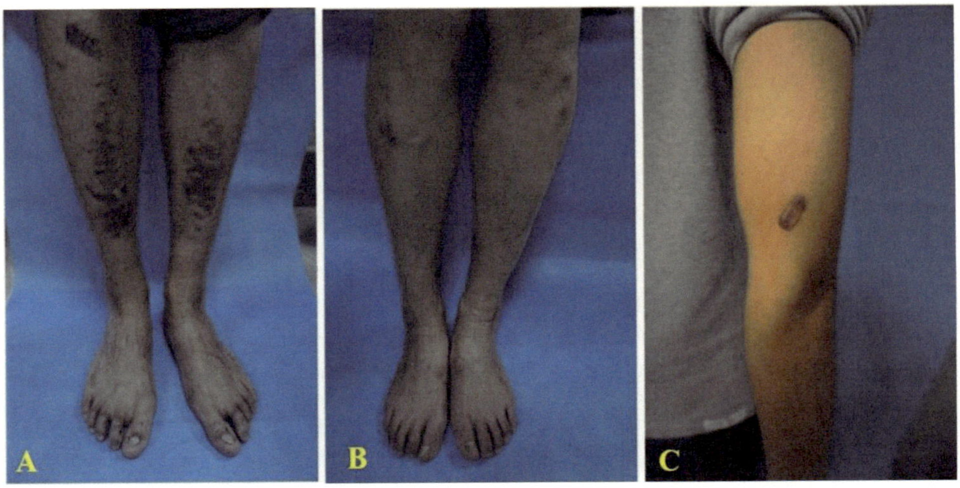

Figure 16.
*Dermatological manifestations of pEDS. A and C were that of the Chinese male with pEDS (**Figure 14**, left panels); B was his mother (**Figure 14**, right panels) with pEDS [69].*

3.4.3 Diagnosis

In the 2017 classification of Ehlers–Danlos syndromes, clinical criteria suggestive for pEDS were defined. Three major criteria and one of the minor criteria must be fulfilled [63].

Major criteria are (1) childhood or adolescence onset severe, intractable periodontitis, (2) thin/atrophic attached gingiva, (3) pretibial pigmented scars, and (4) a first-degree relative in family who also meets pEDS clinical criteria.

Minor pEDS diagnostic criteria include easy bruising, joint hypermobility (typically distal joints), skin hyperextensibility and fragility, atypical scarring, proneness to infections, hernias, marfanoid facial features, acrogeria, and prominent vasculature.

A clinical diagnosis of pEDS should be confirmed with genetic testing. pEDS was caused by dominant gain of function mutations in *C1R* or *C1S*.

3.4.4 Treatment

There is no curative treatment for pEDS. Conservative treatments were offered including oral hygiene instruction, periodontal maintenance about every 3 months or more frequently as the dentist/periodontist sees fit, systemic antibiotics, removable dental prostheses, skin sparing, injury or wound avoidance, emotional support. pEDS patients were reported to have high risk of peri-implant disease also so intense implant maintenance is mandatory [63, 64, 70].

3.4.5 Genetic counseling

Transmission is autosomal dominant. Genetic counseling should be offered to the parents of an affected individual informing them of the 50% chance that their offspring could inherit the disease.

3.4.6 Prognosis

Despite meticulous dental care, pEDS patients eventually become edentulous at an early age (mean age 20 years; range 14–48 years). Life expectancy of pEDS individual is otherwise same as their unaffected counterparts [63, 64, 66].

3.5 Hypophosphatasia

Hypophosphatasia (HPP) is a rare, systemic, genetic, metabolic disease with a deficiency in tissue nonspecific alkaline phosphatase (ALP) activity resulting in the extracellular accumulation of its substrates [71]. The clinical presentation of HPP can vary considerably between individuals and includes skeletal problems, muscle weakness, ambulatory difficulties, pain, and dental, neurologic, and renal manifestations. The first case of HPP was reported by the Canadian pediatrician John Campbell Rathbun in 1948 as a new developmental anomaly. The prevalence of HPP was estimated as 1 in 100,000 live births in the Toronto area in Canada; In Europe, the prevalence of severe cases is estimated as 1 in 300,000 [72].

3.5.1 Etiology and pathogenesis

HPP is mainly caused by alkaline phosphatase, biomineralization associated (*ALPL*) gene mutations. At least 300 *ALPL* gene mutations have been reported. The gene encoding tissue non-specific alkaline phosphatase (TNSALP) or the alkaline phosphatase expressed in bone/kidney/liver is located on chromosome 1. The HPP mutation sites are heterogenous and the disease can be inherited in an autosomal dominant or recessive manner. Inactivating mutation of *ALPL* gene leads to decrease TNSALP, which in turn causes accumulation of extracellular TNSALP substrates like phosphoethanolamine, pyridoxal-5′-phosphate and pyrophosphate hence inhibiting hydroxyapatite formation in physicochemical fashion. At the same time, extracellular pyrophosphate induces osteopontin production and the latter inhibits formation of hydroxyapatite. The aforementioned are the main mechanisms that causes early tooth loss and abnormal bone mineralization in HPP patients [73, 74].

3.5.2 Clinical manifestations

HPP is classified into six forms depending on the onset age and the clinical severity [72]. As shown in **Table 4**, HPP may exhibit perinatal presentation: a severe and possibly fatal infantile form within 6 months of life; milder childhood disease: presenting at childhood or late adolescence as early as 6–24 months; adult disease: a form of odontohypophosphatasia; or a rare benign prenatal form. Among them, odontohypophosphatasia, the least severe form without skeletal ailment, characterized by taurodontism with absence of root cementum. The latter is associated with inadequate/ineffective attachment apparatus of the tooth hence giving raise to premature exfoliation of deciduous teeth (**Figures 17** and **18**).

3.5.3 Diagnosis

HPP diagnosis is based on clinical manifestations, laboratory assays, and genetic testing. Clinical manifestations and low alkaline phosphatase activity can confirm a diagnosis of HPP [72, 75]:

1. Prominent clinical symptoms of HPP include the following: i) Dental: premature or nontraumatic tooth loss with the root intact; ii) Skeletal: severe hypomineralization, skeletal deformities, craniosynostosis, rachitic chest, rickets, bowing, short stature, osteomalacia, bone pain, frequent fractures; iii) Muscular: muscle weakness, hypotonia, muscular/joint pain, waddling gait, difficulty walking. Other Symptoms may include: i) Respiratory: respiratory insufficiency, respiratory failure; ii) Neurologic: vitamin B_6-responsive

Clinical Form	Inheritance	Age of onset	Clinical features	Dental defects	Prognosis
Perinatal lethal	AR	In utero and at birth	Most severe form; Nearly always fatal soon after birth	N/A	Lethal
Benign prenatal	AD	In utero	Mild postnatal course with spontaneous improvement in bony symptoms	N/A	Benign
Infantile	AR	<6 months	Respiratory failure within weeks to months of birth	Premature loss of deciduous teeth	Mostly lethal
Child-hood	AR (frequent) or AD (rare)	≥ 6 months-18 years	Wide range of severities: Short stature Bone pain/fractures	Premature loss of deciduous teeth	Benign
Adult	AR or AD	≥ 18 years	Stress fractures: metatarsal, tibia Chronic bone pain	H/O premature deciduous tooth loss	Benign
Odonto-hypo-phosphatasia	AR or AD	Before 4–5 years	Loss of alveolar bone	Early Exfoliation of primary teeth. Hypoplastic Cementum, dentin. Enlarged pulp chambers. Dental caries	Benign

AD, autosomal dominant; AR, autosomal recessive.

Table 4.
Clinical forms of hypophosphatasia (HPP).

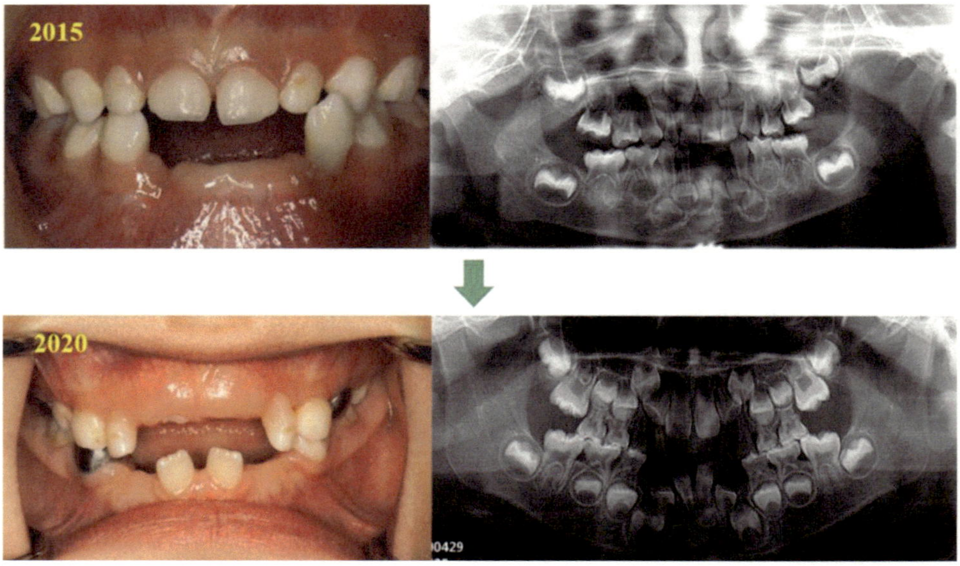

Figure 17.
Oral manifestations of a boy at 2- (upper panels)/7-years old (lower panels) with hypophosphatasia (HPP), odontohypophosphatasia form.

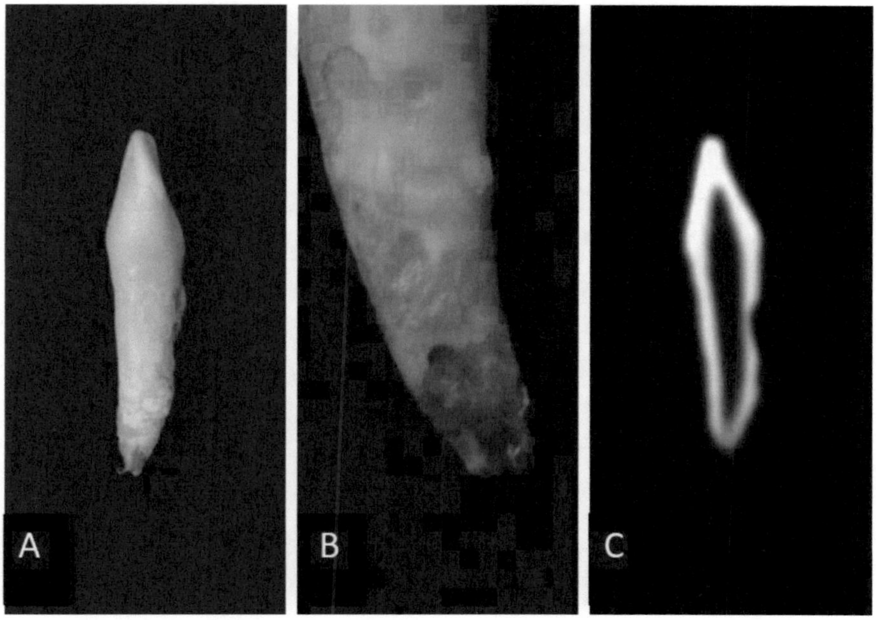

Figure 18.
Exfoliated deciduous teeth showing intact root with distinct lack of cementum. Clinical view of the exfoliated mandibular right lateral incisor (tooth 82): the intact root with hypoplasia of the cementum and external apical root resorption (A, B), Cone beam CT image of the tooth 82 (C) with enlargement of the pulp chamber and root canal.

seizures, increased intracranial pressure; iii) Renal: hypercalciuria, nephrocalcinosis, renal damage; iv) Growth: failure to thrive, delayed or missed motor milestone, short stature.

2. Laboratory assays: Low ALP is the biochemical hallmark of hypophosphatasia. When clinical manifestations of HPP are present, checking for low ALP activity can confirm a diagnosis. In patients with a family history of HPP, testing for low ALP at the first presentation of clinical symptoms may be appropriate. **Figure 19** shows the results of age- and gender-adjusted alkaline phosphatase activity.

3. Genetic testing: *TNAP* gene mutations screening is crucial to HPP diagnosis confirmation especially when biochemical and clinical data appear ambiguous. The genetic test is also a useful prerequisite for genetic counseling for families affected by severe HPP who are in need for molecular prenatal diagnosis.

HPP is often misdiagnosed because its signs and symptoms can overlap with those of other disorders, including nutritional rickets, X-linked hypophosphatemic rickets, and osteogenesis imperfecta. ALP can differentiate HPP from nutritional rickets and other metabolic disorders (**Table 5**).

3.5.4 Treatment

HPP treatment varies depending on its stage and classification and focus on supportive therapy to minimize disease-related systemic manifestations [72, 75, 77], including: i) Vitamin B6 for seizures in affected patients; ii) Surgery to relieve intracranial pressure or repair fractures, experts recommend managing pseudo-fractures secondary to hypophosphatasia by internal fixation with a load-bearing

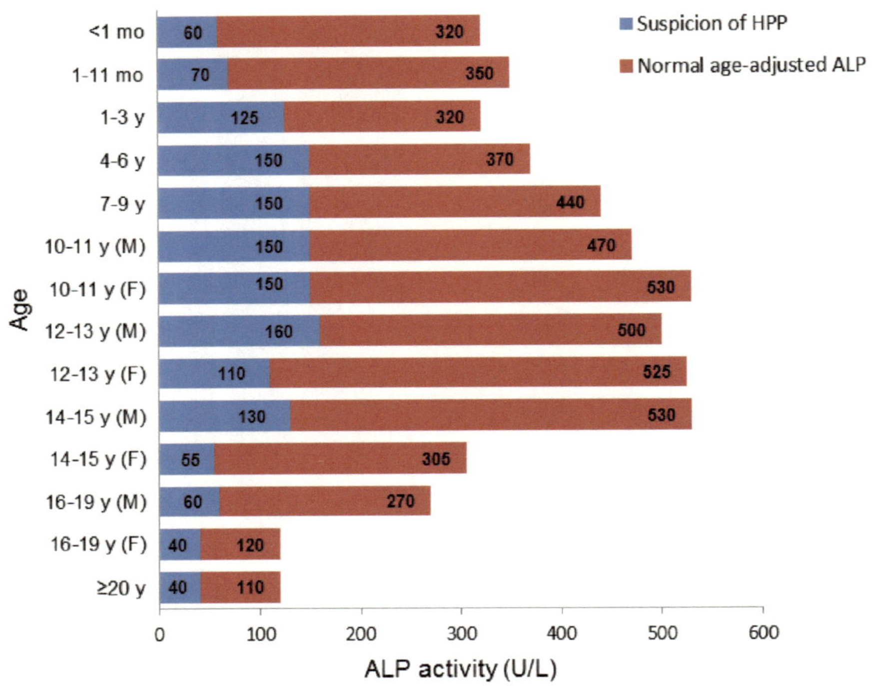

Figure 19.
Age and gender adjusted alkaline phosphatase (ALP) reference ranges.

Biochemical Indicators	**Disorder**			
	HPP	**Nutritional rickets**	**x-linked hypophosphatemic rickets**	**Osteogenesis imperfecta**
ALP	↓	↑	↑	normal
PLP	↑ or normal	—	↓	—
Calcium	↑ or normal	↓	normal	normal
Phosphate	↓ or normal	↓	↓	normal
Parathyroid hormone	↓ or normal	↓	↓ or normal	normal
Vitamin D	normal	↓	↓ or normal	normal

Table 5.
Alkaline phosphatase (ALP) level differentiating hypophosphatasia (HPP) from other metabolic disorders [76].

device without removal; iii) Pain management, such as NSAIDs. High-dose vitamin D, calcium supplements, and bisphosphonates should not be given when HPP is suspected, as they have been shown to exacerbate symptoms of HPP; iv) Dental care to preserve primary dentition. It is often needed to extract primary teeth with high mobility, but on the permanent dentition it is suggested to follow a more conservative therapy and try to keep all teeth as long as possible.

A causal enzyme therapy replacement with asfotase-alfa was approved by FDA in 2015. Asfotase-alfa improves respiratory insufficiency, bone mineralization, and long-term survival, and has a very good safety profile [75, 78].

3.5.5 Genetic counseling

Severe forms of HPP (perinatal and infantile) are inherited via an autosomal recessive fashion, while milder HPP appears to transmit in autosomal recessive or autosomal dominant manner. The risk of severe HPP recurrence therefore, is considered at around 25% while moderate HPP transmission could be 25% (recessive transmission), 50% (dominant transmission) or varying (usually <50%) due to the variable expressivity of dominant HPP forms [71, 72].

3.5.6 Prognosis

The perinatal HPP is often lethal within days if not weeks after birth with approximately 50% of the affected infants succumbing to respiratory complications. Report on prolonged case survival was lacking for infantile or childhood HPP. Patients affected by adult HPP or odontohypophosphatasia, on the other hand, were expected to enjoy a normal lifespan [71, 72, 75].

4. Conclusion

Periodontal disease and especially periodontitis are often the major clinical characteristic of these genetic disorders. In light of the fact periodontal disease may be the first detectable sign of an undiagnosed genetic disorder and/or indicator for the latter's activity progression, oral health professions shall acquire essential knowledge and be cognizant regarding the rare occasions that these diseases could be encountered. In this chapter, we discussed some genetic disorders associated to periodontal disease, we hope this work can help dental practitioners to be familiar with these genetic disorders and their negative impacts on the periodontal tissues hence poor oral/periodontal health of the affected.

Acknowledgements

We thank all the patients in this work, Prof. Houxuan Li and Dr. Juan Liu from department of periodontology, Nanjing Stomatological Hospital, Medical School of Nanjing University. This work was supported in part by the Nanjing Medical Science and Technology Development Program (YKK18121 to JW), the Natural Science Foundation of Jiangsu Province (BK20200149 to JW), and the Health and Medical Research Fund, Hong Kong Special Administrative Region, China (02132216 to WKL).

Conflict of interest

The authors declare no conflict of interest.

Author details

Juan Wu[1], Wai Keung Leung[2*] and Weibin Sun[1*]

1 Department of Periodontology, Nanjing Stomatological Hospital, Medical School of Nanjing University, Nanjing, China

2 Faculty of Dentistry, The University of Hong Kong, Hong Kong SAR, China

*Address all correspondence to: ewkleung@hku.hk and wbsun@nju.edu.cn

References

[1] Clark WB, Löe H. Mechanisms of initiation and progression of periodontal disease. Periodontol 2000. 1993;2:72–82. doi:10.1111/j.1600-0757.1993.tb00221.x

[2] Nanci A, Bosshardt DD. Structure of periodontal tissues in health and disease. Periodontol 2000. 2006;40:11–28. doi:10.1111/j.1600-0757.2005.00141.x

[3] Armitage GC. Development of a classification system for periodontal diseases and conditions. Ann Periodontol. 1999;4(1):1–6. doi:10.1902/annals.1999.4.1.1

[4] Chapple ILC, Mealey BL, Van Dyke TE, et al. Periodontal health and gingival diseases and conditions on an intact and a reduced periodontium: Consensus report of workgroup 1 of the 2017 World Workshop on the Classification of Periodontal and Peri-Implant Diseases and Conditions. J Clin Periodontol. 2018;45 Suppl 20:S68-S77. doi:10.1111/jcpe.12940

[5] Papapanou PN, Sanz M, Buduneli N, et al. Periodontitis: Consensus report of workgroup 2 of the 2017 World Workshop on the Classification of Periodontal and Peri-Implant Diseases and Conditions. J Clin Periodontol. 2018;45 Suppl 20:S162-S170. doi:10.1111/jcpe.12946

[6] Albandar JM, Susin C, Hughes FJ. Manifestations of systemic diseases and conditions that affect the periodontal attachment apparatus: Case definitions and diagnostic considerations. J Clin Periodontol. 2018;45 Suppl 20:S171-S189. doi:10.1111/jcpe.12947

[7] Bird LM, Tan WH. Treatment of genetic disorders-A vision coming into focus. Am J Med Genet C Semin Med Genet. 2016;172(4):311–312. doi:10.1002/ajmg.c.31535

[8] Pizzo G, Lo Re D, Piscopo MR, Pizzo I, Giuliana G. Genetic disorders and periodontal health: a literature review. Med Sci Monit. 2009;15(8):RA167-RA178.

[9] Hanisch M, Hoffmann T, Bohner L, et al. Rare Diseases with Periodontal Manifestations. Int J Environ Res Public Health. 2019;16(5):867. doi:10.3390/ijerph16050867

[10] Meyle J, Gonzáles JR. Influences of systemic diseases on periodontitis in children and adolescents. Periodontol 2000. 2001;26:92–112. doi:10.1034/j.1600-0757.2001.2260105.x

[11] Pinna R, Cocco F, Campus G, et al. Genetic and developmental disorders of the oral mucosa: Epidemiology; molecular mechanisms; diagnostic criteria; management. Periodontol 2000. 2019;80(1):12–27. doi:10.1111/prd.12261

[12] Cheng RHW, Yiu CKY, Leung WK. Oral health in individuals with Down Syndrome. *In*: Dey S ed. Prenatal Diagnosis and Screening for Down Syndrome. InTech - Open Access Publisher, Rijeka, Croatia, 2011. Part 2. Dentistry and skeletal features. Chapter 5, pp. 59–76. ISBN 978-953-307-355-2. doi: 10.5772/17973

[13] Gawron K, Łazarz-Bartyzel K, Potempa J, Chomyszyn-Gajewska M. Gingival fibromatosis: clinical, molecular and therapeutic issues. Orphanet J Rare Dis. 2016;11:9. doi:10.1186/s13023-016-0395-1

[14] Boutiou E, Ziogas IA, Giannis D, Doufexi AE. Hereditary gingival fibromatosis in children: a systematic review of the literature. Clin Oral Investig. doi:10.1007/s00784-020-03682-x.

[15] Costa CRR, Braz SV, de Toledo IP, et al. Syndromes with gingival

fibromatosis: A systematic review. Oral Dis. doi:10.1111/odi.13369.

[16] Hart TC, Pallos D, Bozzo L, et al. Evidence of genetic heterogeneity for hereditary gingival fibromatosis. J Dent Res. 2000;79(10):1758–1764. doi: 10.1177/00220345000790100501

[17] Xiao S, Bu L, Zhu L, et al. A new locus for hereditary gingival fibromatosis (GINGF2) maps to 5q13-q22. Genomics. 2001;74(2):180–185. doi: 10.1006/geno.2001.6542

[18] Ye X, Shi L, Cheng Y, et al. A novel locus for autosomal dominant hereditary gingival fibromatosis, GINGF3, maps to chromosome 2p22.3-p23.3. Clin Genet. 2005;68(3):239–244. doi:10.1111/j.1399-0004.2005.00488.x.

[19] Zhu Y, Zhang W, Huo Z, et al. A novel locus for maternally inherited human gingival fibromatosis at chromosome 11p15. Hum Genet. 2007; 121(1):113–123. doi:10.1007/s00439-006-0283-1

[20] Xiao S, Wang X, Qu B, et al. Refinement of the locus for autosomal dominant hereditary gingival fibromatosis (GINGF) to a 3.8-cM region on 2p21. Genomics. 2000;68(3): 247–252. doi:10.1006/geno.2000.6285

[21] Hart TC, Zhang Y, Gorry MC, et al. A mutation in the SOS1 gene causes hereditary gingival fibromatosis type 1. Am J Hum Genet. 2002;70(4):943–954. doi:10.1086/339689

[22] Bayram Y, White JJ, Elcioglu N, et al. REST Final-Exon-Truncating Mutations Cause Hereditary Gingival Fibromatosis. Am J Hum Genet. 2017; 101(1):149–156. doi:10.1016/j.ajhg.2017.06.006

[23] Wu J, Chen D, Huang H, et al. A Novel Gene *ZNF862* Causes Hereditary Gingival Fibromatosis. medRxiv. 2020; Corpus ID: 218034530.

[24] Gawron K, Ochała-Kłos A, Nowakowska Z, et al. TIMP-1 association with collagen type I overproduction in hereditary gingival fibromatosis. Oral Dis. 2018;24(8):1581–1590. doi:10.1111/odi.12938

[25] Roman-Malo L, Bullon B, de Miguel M, Bullon P. Fibroblasts Collagen Production and Histological Alterations in Hereditary Gingival Fibromatosis. Diseases. 2019;7(2):39. doi:10.3390/diseases7020039

[26] Martelli-Junior H, Cotrim P, Graner E, Sauk JJ, Coletta RD. Effect of transforming growth factor-beta1, interleukin-6, and interferon-gamma on the expression of type I collagen, heat shock protein 47, matrix metalloproteinase (MMP)-1 and MMP-2 by fibroblasts from normal gingiva and hereditary gingival fibromatosis. J Periodontol. 2003;74(3):296–306. doi: 10.1902/jop.2003.74.3.296

[27] Coletta RD, Graner E. Hereditary gingival fibromatosis: a systematic review. J Periodontol. 2006;77(5):753–764. doi:10.1902/jop.2006.050379

[28] Zhou M, Xu L, Meng HX. Diagnosis and treatment of a hereditary gingival fibromatosis case. Chin J Dent Res. 2011; 14(2):155–158.

[29] Roman-Malo L, Bullon B, de Miguel M, Bullon P. Fibroblasts Collagen Production and Histological Alterations in Hereditary Gingival Fibromatosis. Diseases. 2019;7(2):39. doi:10.3390/diseases7020039

[30] Ramer M, Marrone J, Stahl B, Burakoff R. Hereditary gingival fibromatosis: identification, treatment, control. J Am Dent Assoc. 1996;127(4): 493–495. doi:10.14219/jada.archive.1996.0242

[31] Papillon MM, Lefèvre P. Deux cas de kératodermie palmaireet plantaire symmétrique (maladie de Meléda) chez

le frèreet la soeur. Coexistence dan les deux cas d'altérations dentaires graves. Bull Soc Fr Derm Syph. 1924;31:82–84.

[32] Haneke E. The Papillon-Lefèvre syndrome: keratosis palmoplantaris with periodontopathy. Report of a case and review of the cases in the literature. Hum Genet. 1979;51(1):1–35. doi: 10.1007/BF00278288

[33] AI Barrak ZM, Alqarni AS, Chalisserry EP, Anil S. Papillon-Lefèvre syndrome: a series of five cases among siblings. J Med Case Rep. 2016;10(1): 260. doi:10.1186/s13256-016-1051-z

[34] Hart TC, Shapira L. Papillon-Lefèvre syndrome. Periodontol 2000. 1994;6:88–100. doi:10.1111/j.1600-0757.1994.tb00029.x

[35] Hart TC, Hart PS, Bowden DW, et al. Mutations of the cathepsin C gene are responsible for Papillon-Lefèvre syndrome. J Med Genet. 1999;36(12): 881–887.

[36] Machado RA, Cuadra-Zelaya FJM, Martelli-Júnior H, et al. Clinical and molecular analysis in Papillon-Lefèvre syndrome. Am J Med Genet A. 2019;179 (10):2124–2131. doi:10.1002/ajmg.a.61285

[37] Toomes C, James J, Wood AJ, et al. Loss-of-function mutations in the cathepsin C gene result in periodontal disease and palmoplantar keratosis. Nat Genet. 1999;23(4):421–424. doi: 10.1038/70525

[38] Wu W, Chen B, Chen X, et al. A novel large deletion combined with a nonsense mutation in a Chinese child with Papillon-Lefèvre syndrome. J Periodontal Res. 2016;51(3):376–380. doi:10.1111/jre.12317

[39] Celenligil H, Kansu E, Ruacan S, Eratalay K. Papillon-Lefèvre syndrome. Characterization of peripheral blood and gingival lymphocytes with monoclonal antibodies. J Clin Periodontol. 1992;19(6):392–397. doi: 10.1111/j.1600-051x.1992.tb00668.x

[40] Batinica M, Stephan A, Steiger J, Tantcheva-Poór I, Eming SA, Fabri M. Stimulus-dependent NETosis by neutrophils from a Papillon-Lefèvre Syndrome patient. J Eur Acad Dermatol Venereol. 2017;31(5):e239-e241. doi: 10.1111/jdv.14004

[41] Velazco CH, Coelho C, Salazar F, Contreras A, Slots J, Pacheco JJ. Microbiological features of Papillon-Lefèvre syndrome periodontitis. J Clin Periodontol. 1999;26(9):622–627. doi: 10.1034/j.1600-051x.1999.260910.x

[42] Upadhyaya JD, Pfundheller D, Islam MN, Bhattacharyya I. Papillon-Lefèvre syndrome: A series of three cases in the same family and a literature review. Quintessence Int. 2017;48(9): 695–700. doi:10.3290/j.qi.a38865

[43] Ullbro C, Crossner CG, Nederfors T, Alfadley A, Thestrup-Pedersen K. Dermatologic and oral findings in a cohort of 47 patients with Papillon-Lefèvre syndrome. J Am Acad Dermatol. 2003;48(3):345–351. doi: 10.1067/mjd.2003.197

[44] Adamski Z, Burchardt D, Pawlaczyk-Kamieńska T, Borysewicz-Lewicka M, Wyganowska-Świątkowska M. Diagnosis of Papillon-Lefèvre syndrome: review of the literature and a case report. Postepy Dermatol Alergol. 2020;37(5):671–676. doi:10.5114/ada.2020.100480

[45] Janjua SA, Iftikhar N, Hussain I, Khachemoune A. Dermatologic, periodontal, and skeletal manifestations of Haim-Munk syndrome in two siblings. J Am Acad Dermatol. 2008;58 (2):339–344. doi:10.1016/j.jaad.2007.08.004

[46] Giannetti L, Apponi R, Dello Diago AM, Jafferany M, Goldust M,

Sadoughifar R. Papillon-Lefèvre syndrome: Oral aspects and treatment. Dermatol Ther. 2020;33(3):e13336. doi: 10.1111/dth.13336

[47] Ullbro C, Crossner CG, Nederfors T, Alfadley A, Thestrup-Pedersen K. Dermatologic and oral findings in a cohort of 47 patients with Papillon-Lefèvre syndrome. J Am Acad Dermatol. 2003;48(3):345–351. doi: 10.1067/mjd.2003.197

[48] Nickles K, Schacher B, Ratka-Krüger P, Krebs M, Eickholz P. Long-term results after treatment of periodontitis in patients with Papillon-Lefèvre syndrome: success and failure. J Clin Periodontol. 2013;40(8):789–798. doi:10.1111/jcpe.12120

[49] Atarbashi-Moghadam F, Atarbashi-Moghadam S, Kazemifard S, Sijanivandi S, Namdari M. Oral rehabilitation of Papillon-Lefèvre syndrome patients by dental implants: a systematic review. J Korean Assoc Oral Maxillofac Surg. 2020;46(4):220–227. doi:10.5125/jkaoms.2020.46.4.220

[50] Newburger PE, Dale DC. Evaluation and management of patients with isolated neutropenia. Semin Hematol. 2013;50(3):198–206. doi:10.1053/j.seminhematol.2013.06.010

[51] Dale DC. Cyclic and chronic neutropenia: an update on diagnosis and treatment. Clin Adv Hematol Oncol. 2011;9(11):868–869.

[52] Dale DC, Bolyard AA, Aprikyan A. Cyclic neutropenia. Semin Hematol. 2002;39(2):89–94. doi:10.1053/shem.2002.31917

[53] Keshwara K, Zanganah Y. Cyclic neutropenia. Br Dent J. 2011;210(5):197–198. doi:10.1038/sj.bdj.2011.151

[54] Palmer SE, Stephens K, Dale DC. Genetics, phenotype, and natural history of autosomal dominant cyclic hematopoiesis. Am J Med Genet. 1996; 66(4):413–422. doi:10.1002/(SICI)1096-8628(19961230)66:4<413::AID-AJMG5>3.0.CO;2-L

[55] Horwitz M, Benson KF, Person RE, Aprikyan AG, Dale DC. Mutations in *ELA2*, encoding neutrophil elastase, define a 21-day biological clock in cyclic haematopoiesis. Nat Genet. 1999;23(4): 433–436. doi:10.1038/70544

[56] Makaryan V, Zeidler C, Bolyard AA, et al. The diversity of mutations and clinical outcomes for *ELANE*-associated neutropenia. Curr Opin Hematol. 2015; 22(1):3–11. doi:10.1097/MOH.0000000000000105

[57] Bellanné-Chantelot C, Clauin S, Leblanc T, et al. Mutations in the *ELA2* gene correlate with more severe expression of neutropenia: a study of 81 patients from the French Neutropenia Register. Blood. 2004;103(11):4119–4125. doi:10.1182/blood-2003-10-3518

[58] Chen Y, Fang L, Yang X. Cyclic neutropenia presenting as recurrent oral ulcers and periodontitis. J Clin Pediatr Dent. 2013;37(3):307–308. doi:10.17796/jcpd.37.3.n8k0111177074828

[59] Dale DC. Cyclic and chronic neutropenia: an update on diagnosis and treatment. Clin Adv Hematol Oncol. 2011;9(11):868–869.

[60] Dale DC, Bolyard A, Marrero T, et al. Long-Term Effects of G-CSF Therapy in Cyclic Neutropenia. N Engl J Med. 2017;377(23):2290–2292. doi: 10.1056/NEJMc1709258

[61] Vanakker O, Callewaert B, Malfait F, Coucke P. The Genetics of Soft Connective Tissue Disorders. Annu Rev Genomics Hum Genet. 2015;16:229–255. doi:10.1146/annurev-genom-090314-050039

[62] Malfait F, Castori M, Francomano CA, Giunta C, Kosho T,

Byers PH. The Ehlers-Danlos syndromes. Nat Rev Dis Primers. 2020;6 (1):64. doi:10.1038/s41572-020-0194-9

[63] Malfait F, Francomano C, Byers P, et al. The 2017 international classification of the Ehlers-Danlos syndromes. Am J Med Genet C Semin Med Genet. 2017;175(1):8–26. doi: 10.1002/ajmg.c.31552

[64] Brady AF, Demirdas S, Fournel-Gigleux S, et al. The Ehlers-Danlos syndromes, rare types. Am J Med Genet C Semin Med Genet. 2017;175(1):70–115. doi:10.1002/ajmg.c.31550

[65] Stewart RE, Hollister DW, Rimoin DL. A new variant of Ehlers Danlos syndrome: an autosomal dominant disorder of fragile skin, abnormal scarring, and generalized periodontitis. Birth Defects Orig Artic Ser. 1977;13(3B):85–93.

[66] Kapferer-Seebacher I, Lundberg P, Malfait F, Zschocke J. Periodontal manifestations of Ehlers-Danlos syndromes: A systematic review. J Clin Periodontol. 2017;44(11):1088–1100. doi:10.1111/jcpe.12807

[67] Kapferer-Seebacher I, Pepin M, Werner R, et al. Periodontal Ehlers-Danlos Syndrome Is Caused by Mutations in C1R and C1S, which Encode Subcomponents C1r and C1s of Complement. Am J Hum Genet. 2016;99(5):1005–1014. doi: 10.1016/j.ajhg.2016.08.019

[68] Gröbner R, Kapferer-Seebacher I, Amberger A, et al. C1R Mutations Trigger Constitutive Complement 1 Activation in Periodontal Ehlers-Danlos Syndrome. Front Immunol. 2019;10: 2537. doi:10.3389/fimmu.2019.02537

[69] Wu J, Yang J, Zhao J, et al. A Chinese family with periodontal Ehlers-Danlos syndrome associated with missense mutation in the C1R gene. J Clin Periodontol. 2018;45(11):1311–1318. doi:10.1111/jcpe.12988

[70] Rinner A, Zschocke J, Schossig A, Gröbner R, Strobl H, Kapferer-Seebacher I. High risk of peri-implant disease in periodontal Ehlers-Danlos Syndrome. A case series. Clin Oral Implants Res. 2018;29(11):1101–1106. doi:10.1111/clr.13373

[71] Whyte MP. Hypophosphatasia: An overview for 2017. Bone. 2017;102:15–25. doi:10.1016/j.bone.2017.02.011

[72] Bianchi ML. Hypophosphatasia: an overview of the disease and its treatment. Osteoporos Int. 2015;26(12): 2743–2757. doi:10.1007/s00198-015-3272-1

[73] Jandl NM, Schmidt T, Rolvien T, et al. Genotype-Phenotype Associations in 72 Adults with Suspected ALPL-Associated Hypophosphatasia. Calcif Tissue Int. 2020;10.1007/s00223-020-00771-7. doi:10.1007/s00223-020-00771-7

[74] Mornet E, Taillandier A, Domingues C, et al. Hypophosphatasia: a genetic-based nosology and new insights in genotype-phenotype correlation. Eur J Hum Genet. 2020; 10.1038/s41431-020-00732-6. doi: 10.1038/s41431-020-00732-6

[75] Khan AA, Josse R, Kannu P, et al. Hypophosphatasia: Canadian update on diagnosis and management. Osteoporos Int. 2019;30(9):1713–1722. doi:10.1007/s00198-019-04921-y

[76] Carpenter TO, Imel EA, Holm IA, et al. A clinician's guide to X-linked hypophosphatemia [published correction appears in J Bone Miner Res. 2015 Feb;30(2):394]. J Bone Miner Res. 2011;26(7):1381–1388. doi:10.1002/jbmr.340

[77] Bangura A, Wright L, Shuler T. Hypophosphatasia: Current Literature for Pathophysiology, Clinical Manifestations, Diagnosis, and Treatment. Cureus. 2020;12(6):e8594.

Published 2020 Jun 13. doi:10.7759/cureus.8594

[78] Bowden SA, Foster BL. Profile of asfotase alfa in the treatment of hypophosphatasia: design, development, and place in therapy. Drug Des Devel Ther. 2018;12:3147–3161. doi:10.2147/DDDT.S154922

Chapter 3

Interdisciplinary Periodontics

Subash Chandra Raj, Shaheda Tabassum, Annuroopa Mahapatra and Kaushik Patnaik

Abstract

Evidence based periodontics has made us understand that most of the patients having various dental or medical treatment requirements require multidisciplinary approach rather than personalised periodontal approach. Periodontal disease may be evident in the periodontal tissue but its onset and progression could be affected by systemic condition also. The intercommunication and liaison between periodontics and endodontics, fixed prosthodontics, implant dentistry, Orthodontics, oral pathology, Aesthetic dentistry, oral & maxillofacial surgery, Paediatric dentistry, gerodontology, radiology, special needs dentistry and general medicine needs to be discussed. Increasing life expectancy, higher quality of Biomaterials used in dentistry and rapid evolution of clinical procedures has led to more demanding patient requests & more complicated treatment choices. It requires holistic management. In this chapter we have made a conscious effort to touch upon various fields of medical science and its relation to periodontics, by which we wish to create a healthy referral protocol, benefiting the general population.

Keywords: Interdisciplinary periodontics, Ortho- perio synergy, periodontal surgery

1. Introduction

The intercommunication and liaison between periodontal tissues/periodontal diseases and endodontics, fixed prosthodontics, implant dentistry,orthodontics, oral pathology, aesthetic dentistry, oral & maxillofacial surgery, paediatric dentistry, gerodontology, radiology, special needs dentistry and general medicine needs to be discussed [1]. Increasing life expectancy, higher quality of Biomaterials used in dentistry and rapid evolution of clinical procedures has led to more demanding patient requests & more complicated treatment choices. It requires holistic management, which frequently mandates clinicians to cooperate in a multidisciplinary approach, in order to fulfil therapeutic objectives and to provide successful treatment concerning functional rehabilitation and aesthetical enhancement [2]. So, clinicians should believe in 'merge to emerge' approach of interdisciplinary Periodontics.

Understanding these interrelationships can improve the clinicians' ability to establish the correct diagnosis, to evaluate the prognosis of affected tooth or teeth and to design and carry out an appropriate treatment according to biological and clinical evidence. Interdisciplinary dentistry can be described as the mutual permeation of various dental specialties accompanied by expansion of the scope of each. The term 'synergy' refers to two or more distinct influences or agents acting together to create an effect greater than that predicted by knowing only the separate

IntechOpen

effects of the individual agents [3]. This definition is applicable to the classic relationships between various specialities in the dentistry that should go hand in hand for the complete well being of the patient. Within modern dentistry, periodontics share an intimate and inseparable relationship with endodontics, orthodontics, Prosthetic dentistry as well as other specialities in multiple aspects including treatment plan, procedure execution, outcome,achievement and maintenance.

Interdisciplinary team work in periodontics is a complex process in which different specialities staff work together to share expertise, knowledge and skills to impact on patient care. Thus the interdisciplinary periodontics can be interpreted as the interaction and interrelationship between periodontist and other dental specialists with harmonious setting & skills sharing common periodontal health goals and practicing concerted physical and mental effort in determining, planning and evaluating patient care [4].

This definition of interdisciplinary periodontics may be more optimistic and aspirational than realistic as it makes several assumptions about the characteristics that a team will possess.

The ten themes identified as the characteristics of a good interdisciplinary team are:

1. Leadership and management - Having a clear leader of the team like a periodontist with a clear direction and management.

2. Communication skill.

3. Personal rewards, training and development - seminar, workshop on interdisciplinary Periodontics.

4. Appropriate resources and procedures - Team members working from the same location, ensuring the appropriate procedures are in place.

5. Appropriate skill mix.

6. Climate - Team culture of trust, valuing contributions, nurturing consensus and need to create an interprofessional atmosphere.

7. Individual characteristics- knowledge, experience, initiatives, knowing strength and weakness etc.

8. Clarity of vision.

9. Quality and outcomes of care.

10. Respecting and understanding roles (**Figure 1**).

All phases of clinical dentistry are intimately related to a common objective. The preservation and maintenance of the natural dentition in health is of prime importance in an integrated interdisciplinary approach to periodontal care. It is logical that periodontal treatment precedes final restorative procedure. Hence, for successful oral rehabilitation of the patient the interdisciplinary approach is required where ideas can be exchanged for the sake of sound oral health [3].

The aim of this chapter is to focus the importance of periodontal examination and periodontist in clinical dental practice and referral in general dental practice. It also describes the intercommunication and liaison between periodontal tissues/

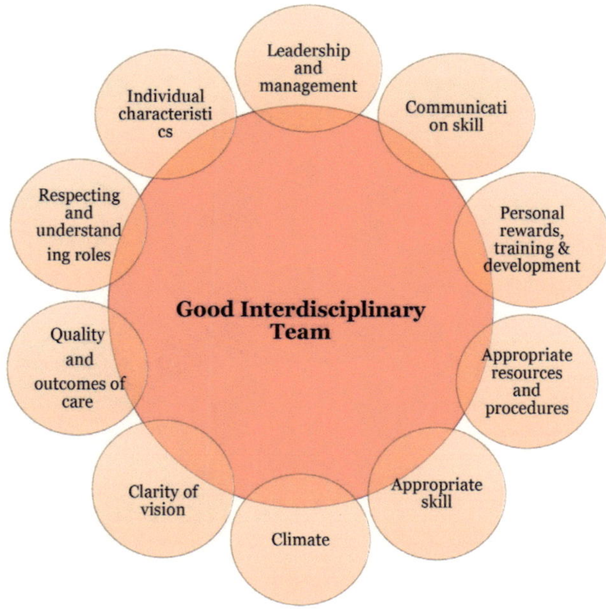

Figure 1.
Schematic diagram for interdisciplinary team.

periodontal diseases and endodontics, fixed prosthodontics, implant dentistry, orthodontics, oral pathology, aesthetic dentistry, oral and maxillofacial surgery, paediatric dentistry, gerodontology, radiology, special needs dentistry and general medicine.

2. Periodontal office as a hub for interdisciplinary approach

2.1 Periodontics and referral in general medicine

The separation of medicine and dentistry is a peculiar historical artefact resulting in medicine being preoccupied with various systems of the body and dentistry being focused on disease and injury of the teeth and its supporting and surrounding structures, jaw and mouth. The professional boundaries are dutifully respected but the distinction has resulted in a poverty of cooperation, greatly inhibiting the synergistic potential. There are numerous diseases that produce both medical and dental complications like chronic kidney disease, cardiovascular disease, endocrine disorders and peripheral vascular disease. These chronic diseases capitulate a huge financial and social burden that necessitate medicine and dentistry to coordinate for achieving a more substantial delivery of care.

Poor oral health affects morbidity more than mortality [5]. Unfortunately, oral health has been a disregarded area of global health and has been registered as low on the sight of National policy makers. Link between oral/periodontal health and systemic health is an established fact now. Despite the awareness regarding the impact of oral health and the increasing attention within public policy, there are barriers preventing access to both basic & specialist dental care. The affordability of dental care and the economic hardships associated with its use presents one of the main barriers to care. The insurance system also determines the frequency with which individuals access dental care. Age is strongly associated with the interval between visits to dentists, despite having increased risk of periodontitis [6].

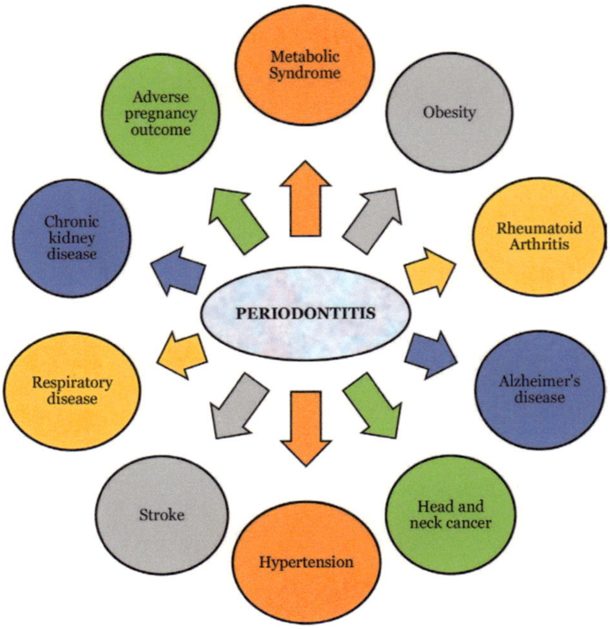

Figure 2.
Periodontitis and its relation to systemic condition.

The impact of periodontal health and the release of inflammatory mediators are not restricted to the cardiovascular and cerebrovascular systems. Periodontal infections influence the initiation and progression of chronic obstructive pulmonary disease and respiratory infections such as pneumonia [7]. Periodontal disease also have been associated with preterm birth and low birth weight baby [8]. Patients with periodontitis have been found to be at increased risk of being in dysmetabolic state,characterised by decreased serum level of high density lipoprotein and mild insulin resistance [9] (**Figure 2**).

There are various common risk factors that explains the link between periodontal diseases and systemic diseases such as age, gender, socio economic status, income, smoking, ethnicity. Therefore, physicians should be well aware of this fact and should identify these risk factors and refer accordingly. These facts should be strengthened in continuing medical education programmes for surgical & physician trainees as well as be put into action into the medical and dental student curriculum. Before referral, the doctor and the dentist should inform the patient why there is reason to be concerned and the importance of managing risk factors. The doctor and dentist should provide a letter of referral for the patient outlining the medical and dental history respectively. The dentist should outline the list of procedures carried out, their impression of prognosis as well as whether there is a requirement for follow-up appointments. Most medical departments should hold regular multidisciplinary team meetings and one possible suggestion would be to include a periodontist.

2.2 The connection between periodontics and oral pathology

The periodontium in health and biofilm induced periodontal infections are very familiar to all oral health professionals including general practitioners and periodontists. The gingiva and buccal mucosa are associated with numerous local and systemic diseases. There are certain rare pathologies that may manifest in soft or hard tissue components of periodontium can be deliberated by by periodontists with oral pathologists and they should act cohesively in aconvenient way so that these pathological conditions are perfectly diagnosed and treated. Not all possible disease processes that affect the gum can be included but it will facilitate a structure to steer the investigations and treatment plan if something abnormal identified.

These are the list of some abnormal lesions of gingiva that can be diagnosed & managed in a timely manner if interdisciplinary approach is followed between periodontist and oral pathologists [1]:

1. Gingival lesions of developmental/ genetic origin
    - Hereditary gingival fibromatosis
    - Ligneous gingivitis
    - Gingival hamartomas
2. Gingival lesions of traumatic origin
    - Peripheral giant cell lesions
    - Brown tumours of hyperparathyroidism
3. Gingival lesions of infectious origin
    - Herpes simplex virus infection
    - HIV infection
4. Gingival lesions considered to have an immunologic origin.
    - Lichen planus
    - Mucous membrane pemphigoid
    - Pemphigus vulgaris
    - Orofacial granulomatosis
    - Langerhans cell histiocytosis
5. Drug induced gingival lesions
    - Drug induced gingival enlargement
    - Drug induced xerostomia
6. Cysts, potentially neoplastic and neoplastic gingival lesions
    - Odontogenic cysts and neoplasms
    - Leukoplakia
    - Squamous cell carcinoma

- Lymphoma
- Peripheral Ameloblastoma
- Malignant melanoma

Lesions of the periodontium may be of a simple local nature or may be an indication of severe local or systemic disease. These patients with such lesions will be referred to periodontists, who will need to have a structured plan to follow when signs and symptoms of gingival pathology persists.

2.3 The interdisciplinary relationship between periodontics and oral and maxillofacial surgery

Oral and maxillofacial surgery and Periodontics are two surgically oriented specialities of dentistry. The education and practice is very contrasting in many countries where an oral and maxillofacial surgeon requires both dental and medical qualification. If restorative procedures limited to the dental hard tissues are excluded, the surgical procedures of the oral cavity include those performed on the oral mucosa, attached gingiva and bone are common to both specialities. The purpose of interdisciplinary approach between these two surgical branches is to highlight some areas of dentistry where patient management could be performed by either speciality and to present some examples where periodontists and oral and maxillofacial surgeons can work closely together to achieve the best possible outcome for the patient.

2.3.1 Surgical exposure of an impacted canine for orthodontics

Impacted maxillary canine can be successfully managed by periodontist as well as oral and maxillofacial surgeon. It mostly depends on the referral pattern of orthodontist and experience of surgeon. Irrespective of who does the treatment, follow up management of the patient is most important. A proper interdisciplinary approach and communication between referring dentist & orthodontist is vital in this. This follow up management for initial 2 to 3 months recall should be individually tailored to the patient.

2.3.2 Removal of mandibular tori

Mandibular lingual tori are common benign osseous growths that may require surgical removal when they are chronically traumatised, affect overall oral hygiene or for prosthodontic reasons. Mandibular tori have also been used as autogenous graft during dental implant surgery [10]. Many times surgeries involving structures close to the floor of the mouth are associated with the complications such as bleeding and airway obstruction [11]. Keeping in mind this complications which may require hospital admission,referral dentist may prefer an oral and maxillofacial surgeon rather than a periodontist.

2.3.3 Autogenous block bone grafting for dental implants

Stability of dental implant is always questionable where there is deficient bone quality and volume [12]. There are many methods of augmenting bone including autogenous onlay bone grafts. Intra oral donor sites for bone harvesting include mandibular ramus, symphysis, retromolar area and maxillary tuberosity. Oral surgeons are more confident in dealing with open bony procedures of high complexity but some periodontists may still wish to continue with the implant treatment of their patient requiring a block bone graft.

Interdisciplinary referral between Periodontist and Oral and Maxillofacial surgeon may be influenced by availability of services in the area, patient preferences and the professional and personal relationships between clinicians. There are many instances where a proper interdisciplinary approach exists between oral and maxillofacial surgeon and periodontist. To identify and appreciate what other specialities have to offer is for the best interest of the patient.

Any patient planned for orthognathic surgery by oral surgeon should be referred to a periodontist for a detailed periodontal examination including assessment of width of keratinized gingiva and thickness of bone, otherwise there will be chances of gingival recession and there should be a close liaison between the restorative dentist and periodontist during the oral rehabilitation phase of any patient with dentofacial deformity.

Early removal of impacted mandibular third molars especially when angulated and in close proximity to the second molar is at increased risk of worsening probing depths and clinical attachment levels. To prevent periodontal defects following mandibular third molar surgery, oral surgeon should work with periodontists for immediate placement of bone graft with and without collagen membrane. When the patient is associated with significant medical problems, periodontist always wish to refer him/her to oral and maxillofacial surgeon. Because of increased risk of morbidity the patient may be best managed in a hospital setting by the oral and maxillofacial surgeon.

2.4 Paediatric dentistry and periodontic interface

It is evidence based that child oral health reflects overall health and also forecasts their condition of oral cavity in youth. Child oral health mostly emphasises on dental caries and is segregated from general health care. So, it has become very crucial to realise the condition of oral tissue and mainly the periodontium in health and disease to facilitate a long lasting oral health in youth.

According to American Academy of Paediatric dentistry, all adolescents and children should perform periodontal screening and recording during their regular dental check-up. It should include colour & shape of gingival margins, plaque visualisation with disclosing agent and height of interproximal bone on radiographs [13]. Regular screening (periodontal screening and recording) is adviced for child and young teens with deciduous and mixed dentition [14]. Such screening helps to find out prior signs and symptoms of destruction of periodontal tissue. With emerging branch of periodontal medicine and established evidence of link between general health and oral health, it has become more important for the physicians and paediatricians to use oral health screening tools, particularly those who do not wish to obtain oral health care facility. Paediatric dentistry and Periodontology should work cohesively to come up with proof, capability and endorsements to ensure that all health professionals will be able to recognise the oral health problems of children.

Periodontal conditions that integrate Pedodontics and Periodontics focus in children:

2.4.1 Dental trauma

The periodontal complex is always prone to be affected by occlusal trauma that can lead to ischemic changes in periodontium. Following periodontal ligament destruction adjoining to alveolar bone, ligament regeneration can occur, and repair-related resorption or resorption ankylosis have also been demonstrated. After occlusal/dental trauma in child and youth, it is important to assess the periodontal staus to have the proper diagnosis and treatment planning that will help to advise the children and their parents of the intended result [15].

2.4.2 Smoking and drug use in adolescence

US centres for disease control in 2012 report, on adulthood and tobacco use, disclosed that 9 out of 10 adult smokers started smoking before 18 years of age [16]. It produces a remarkable influence on risk of having periodontal disease. Therefore health professionals should utilise regular questioning and furnish particulars to the young patients regarding the bad effects of smoking on periodontal health. Regular Smoking corresponds with gingival inflammation and repeated bleeding on probing [17]. It is important to identify history of smoking and seek to reduce the risk of significant impact of smoking on periodontal health.

2.4.3 Overweight, obesity, metabolic syndrome and diabetes

Child and young adults with obesity, overweight and pre diabetic conditions have been reported to have increased prevalence of dental caries and periodontal disease [18].

2.4.4 Respiratory diseases

Recent reports advocate that bacteria from oral cavity can be accountable for many respiratory diseases like aspiration pneumonia [19]. There is a chance for Pedodontists and Periodontists to promote impressive and useful methods to prop up oral health in children and young people with chronic obstructive pulmonary disease (**Figure 3**).

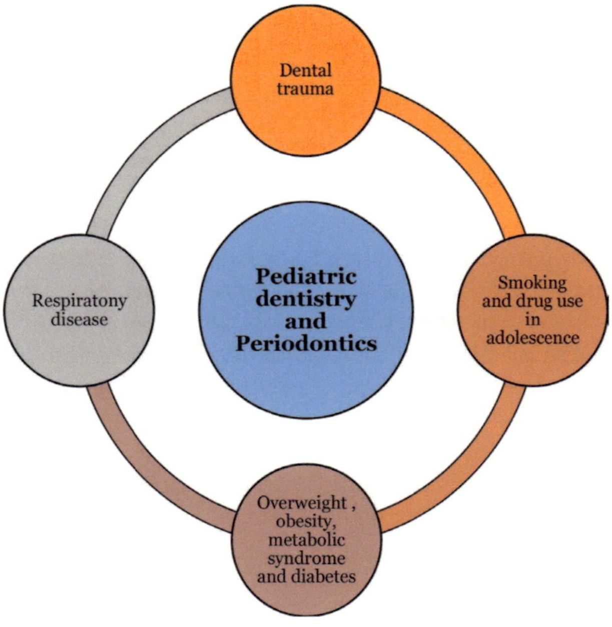

Figure 3.
Periodontal disease as a risk factor for systemic condition.

It is becoming more evident that there is a direct link between periodontal health and general health. Identifying oral health problems during early childhood would draw a preventive attention on periodontal tissues. Keeping this in mind pedodontist and periodontist can work cohesively to ameliorate durable oral health outcomes for children and adolescents.

2.5 Ortho–perio synergy

The term 'synergy' refers to two or more distinct influences or agents acting together to create an effect greater than that predicted by knowing only the separate effects of the individual agents. This definition is applicable to the classic relationship between orthodontics and periodontics specialities in treating patients [20, 21]. No matter how talented an orthodontist is, a magnificent orthodontic correction can be destroyed by a failure to recognise periodontal susceptibility.

The interrelationship between Orthodontics and Periodontics often resembles symbiosis [22]. In many cases, periodontal health is improved by orthodontic tooth movement, whereas orthodontic tooth movement is often facilitated by periodontal therapy. A multidisciplinary approach is often required for the correction of complex dentoalveolar problems in patients and this can be better explained by ortho-perio integration.

Periodontal disease is not necessarily a contraindication to orthodontic treatment provided that the condition has been stabilised; however loss of alveolar bone and soft tissue architecture may pose considerable challenges to oral rehabilitation. It has been suggested that adjunct orthodontic treatment may play an important role in developing the optimal base needed for re-establishing an aesthetic and functional dentition in these cases.

Orthodontic patients can be classified into three categories-

1. Patients with good oral health

2. Patients with periodontal disease and /or loss of permanent teeth.

3. Patients with severe skeletal discrepancies.

Patients belonging to the second category needs a multi-disciplinary approach requiring periodontist and orthodontist. For treating these type of patients both specialists should be called for during treatment planning and follow up management.

2.5.1 Evaluation of orthodontic patients for periodontal problem

Though bleeding on probing is usually a sign of active periodontal disease, on a practical note absence of bleeding on probing is a superior foresee criteria of periodontal health. In other way, even though there is presence of pocket depth, an absence of bleeding on probing can be used as a test of healthy gums. Bleeding on probing is usually checked by inserting a graduated metallic or plastic probe into gingival sulcus at an agreeable range of force between 10 to 20 gms. Patients requiring orthodontic treatment or under active orthodontic therapy should be informed of this persistent bleeding on probing and should be cautioned that they are at risk of periodontal disease and thus they need to consult a periodontist.

Researches have indicated the gravity of complete periodontal examination with a graduated periodontal probe, 6 sites per tooth for an extensive interpretation of periodontal status mostly bleeding on probing and probing pocket depth in orthodontic patients [23, 24].

2.5.2 Orthodontic treatment and its effect on periodontium

It has been widely believed that appropriately applied orthodontic forces do not damage the periodontium. However, insufficient width of attached gingiva is widely believed to be a predisposing factor for gingival recession. Orthodontic treatment and retention phase may be a risk factor for labial gingival recession. After orthodontic treatment with fixed appliance, the incidence increases from 7% at the end of treatment to 20% at 2 yrs. after treatment and to 38% at 5 years after treatment [25]. Alveolar bone dehiscence is also a predisposing factor for gingival recession.

Steiner et al. suggested that tension in the marginal tissue created by the orthodontic forces could be an important factor in causing gingival recession. Thickness of gingival tissue (Gingival biotype) at pressure side is an indicator of possible gingival recession [26].

Greenbaum et al. studied the effects of slow and rapid maxillary expansion on periodontium. They concluded that patients subjected to rapid maxillary expansion showed significantly lesser bone relative to the cementoenamel junction when compared to patients treated with slow expansion [27].

Erkan et al. observed that gingival margin and mucogingival junction moved in the same direction along with teeth when orthodontic intrusion is done. Extrusion also produces gingival margin and mucogingival junction movement in same direction as the extruded teeth resulting in reduction of sulcus depth without reduction in the width of attached gingiva [28].

2.5.3 Orthodontic treatment as an adjunct to periodontal therapy

Various orthodontic treatments such as up righting, intrusion and rotation are performed to correct pathologically migrated teeth that control further periodontal breakdown, improve oral function and provide acceptable aesthetics. These procedures should be performed only after stabilising active periodontal disease.

Despite of inconsistent relation between malocclusion and periodontal disease, connection of crowded or malposed teeth permit the patient better access to clean all the surfaces of his/her teeth. Food impactions are also reduced or eliminated by the creation of proper arch form and proximal contact [29, 30].

Orthodontic uprighting of the tilted molars has several advantages: the distal movement of teeth allows the deposition of alveolar bone on the mesial defect, thereby eliminating the gingival folding and plaque retentive area on mesial side [31].

Orthodontic extrusion of teeth may be indicated for shallowing out intraosseous defects and for increasing the clinical crown length of single rooted teeth. Orthodontic intrusion has been recommended for teeth with horizontal bony defect or infrabony pockets [32].

The hemiseptal defects or one wall defect can be eliminated using uprighting, extrusion and levelling of the bone defect [31]. Bodily movement of the tooth into an intrabony defect has been believed to carry the bone along with the tooth, that results in improvement of defect. This will ameliorate neighbouring tooth position prior to placing implant or replacing the tooth. If the tooth is supraerupted with osseous defect, intrusion and levelling of the bony defect can help to eliminate these problems.

Deepa outlined the utility of orthodontic soft aligners in relocating a periodontally compormised tooth. Light and intermittent forces generated by the soft aligner allow regeneration of tissue during tooth movement [33].

Complaisance of patient, encouragement and oral hygiene maintenance will facilitate to identify the perfect time to initiate adjunctive orthodontic treatment.

If enough confirmation of complete resolve of inflammation is achieved then orthodontic treatment can be started six months after active periodontal therapy.

2.5.4 Periodontics as an adjunct to orthodontic treatment

In many instances a consistent and aesthetically appreciable result may not be accomplished with orthodontic therapy without concomitant periodontal treatment. For example, a papilla or papilla penetrating type of frenal attachment is thought to be an etiologic factor of midline diastema. Frenectomy is performed for them because the fibres are thought to obstruct the mesial migration of incisors. However, when to perform frenectomy has been a debatable issue.

Vanarsdall pointed out that, excision of a maxillary labial frenum should be hold up until after orthodontic treatment unless it obstructs space closure or associated with pain or trauma. The best time to do frenectomy is after your orthodontist has closed the space & before placing the retainer. Scar tissue that forms between the teeth as a result of surgery might actually make the space harder to close during treatment and force the teeth back apart afterwards [34].

Miller's technique of frenectomy is best suited for orthodontic cases. Post operatively on healing, there is a continuous collagenous band of gingiva across the midline that gives a bracing effect than the 'scar' tissue, thus preventing an orthodontic relapse. The transseptal fibres are not disrupted surgically and so there is no loss of interdental papilla [35]. Retention of orthodontically achieved tooth rotation is a problem that has always plagued orthodontist. Circumferential supracrestal fibrotomy (CSF) or Pericision is a procedure that is frequently used to enhance post treatment stability [36].

It is suggested that some cases of potential or actual mucogingival problems may be improved by tooth movement. Since orthodontic and conservative periodontal therapy may induce changes in the character and level of attached gingiva, soft tissue grafts may be unnecessary. However if periodontal biotype is thin, soft tissue grafts may be required before orthodontic treatment, otherwise orthodontic tooth movement may result in gingival recession.

In case of angular defects, regenerative procedures may be performed after orthodontic treatment except in cases where the remaining bone support is not sufficient for anchorage. Bony topography may improve after orthodontic treatment and the osseous grafts placed may be displaced during orthodontic tooth movement. If osseous grafts are to be placed prior to orthodontic treatment then 6–8 months of waiting period is necessary to start orthodontic treatment.

2.5.5 Periodontally accelerated osteogenic orthodontics or Wilkodontics

The biology behind Periodontally accelerated osteogenic orthodontics is the regional acceleratory phenomenon (RAP). It has several advantages such as reduction of treatment time, facilitates expansion of dental arch, produces less root resorption rate compared to normal tooth movement, improved post orthodontic stability and slower relapse tendency [37].

It is a corticotomy facilitated technique which involves a full thickness labial and lingual flap elevation accompanied by selective corticomy followed by placement of bone graft material, surgical closure and orthodontic force application.

Piezosurgery assisted orthodontics is a new minimally invasive surgical procedure, in which microincisions are performed on buccal/labial gingiva that allows the piezoelectric knife to give osseous cuts to the buccal cortical plate and initiate RAP. This procedure also maintains the clinical benefit of the bone or soft tissue grafting along with tunnel approach. Compared to classical corticotomy procedure, piezocision has added advantage of being minimally invasive, safe and less traumatic to the patient. In the recent years, because of the increased number of adults seeking orthodontic treatment, orthodontists frequently face patients with periodontal disease. Adult patient must undergo regular oral hygiene performance and periodontal maintenance in order to maintain healthy gingival tissue during active orthodontic therapy. Since orthodontic therapy and.

periodontal health shares a close relation, an understanding of the ortho-perio relationship helps in executing the best possible outcomes in needy patients.

2.6 Prostho - perio interrelationship - PROSPER

Periodontics and Prosthodontics hold one of the powerful & close connections of all disciplines of modern dentistry. Healthy periodontium is vital for long term success of restorations, on the other hand defect in prosthesis may give rise to progression of periodontal disease [38].

2.6.1 Restorative consideration that impact the periodontium

The relationship between periodontal health and restoration of teeth is intimate and inseparable. For restoration to survive long term, the periodontium must remain healthy so that the teeth are maintained [39]. Following considerations are to be taken care:

1. Restoration contour and contact areas

2. Margin adaptation and defects

3. Location of margin

4. Role of Provisional restoration

5. Design of fixed and removable partial dentures

6. Occlusal function

7. Prosthetic and restorative materials and alloy hypersensitivity

8. Iatrogenic damage from restorative procedures

Clinical longevity of any prosthesis is directly related to achieving proper restorative contours [40]. It is the function of the axial form of teeth to afford protection and stimulation to marginal periodontium. Schluger et al. felt that cervical bulge (>0.5 mm than cementoenamel junction) overprotects the microbial plaque. They advocated flat contours, not fat contours [41]. Overcontouring is potentially more detrimental to periodontium than undercontouring.

Scientific data indicates that even clinically successful crowns have margins that are open and average opening is about 100 nm, which tends to accumulate bacterial plaque [42]. Roughness of the tooth-restoration interface forms scratches on the surface of carefully polished acrylic and ceramic crowns. Inadequate marginal fit of the restoration, dissolution and disintegration of the luting material causes crater formation between the preparation and restoration and inflammation of gingiva [43].

Eissman et.al's design criteria for fixed partial dentures state that crown margins should be placed on tooth surfaces that are fully exposed to cleansing action, preferably supragingival or slightly into sulcus [44]. Vigorous tooth brushing was effective upto 0.7 mm below the gingival margin, suggesting that the submarginal extension of restoration should be limited to no more than this distance. Restorative requirements frequently necessitate subgingival margin placement in order to gain resistance or retention form to alter tooth contour, subgingival caries, furcation involvement, to hide the tooth restoration interface or have contacts that need to be lengthened apically to avoid black triangles.

Current trends favour equigingival margin over older concepts of subgingival margin for crowns, which are kinder to periodontium. Furthermore, advances with emerging materials like translucent restorative materials, adhesive dentistry and resin cements promote polished margins that aesthetically blend with the tooth for a healthy tooth-restorative interface even when placed equigingivally [45].

Provisional restorations are needed to protect the prepared teeth to reduce the sensitivity of the vital abutments and to prevent tooth migration. Provisionals should have good marginal fit and polish. This prevents plaque accumulation and related inflammatory gingival overgrowth or recession.

A bridge should be designed to minimise the accumulation of dental plaque and food debris and to maximise access for cleansing by patient. It should also provide embrasures for the passage of food and protection of gingival crevices [46]. Stein concluded that pontic design is more important than the material used in pontic construction [47]. The undersurface of pontics in fixed bridges should barely touch the mucosa. The 'modified ridge lap' pontic has pinpoint, pressure free contact on the facial slope of ridge and all surfaces should be convex, smooth and highly glazed or polished. The sanitary pontic is most hygienic but ovate pontic combines both aesthetic and hygiene. Crowns that are placed on upper molars that have undergone root resection must be contoured in a specific way to ensure that the patient has access to oral hygiene measures. The gingival embrasure form created in the restoration must be fluted into these areas so that the surfaces can be accessed by an interdental brush, a knife edge or chamfer margin is indicated.

Occlusal discrepancies in a restoration appear to be a significant risk factor that contributes to more rapid periodontal destruction. Cantilever design often result in fracture of casting and periodontal inflammation around abutment tooth.

2.6.2 The impacts of periodontal/implant health on prosthetic therapy

Prior to treatment plan, tooth prognosis should be addressed both on individual tooth and the overall dentition. While assessing individual tooth prognosis it is important to identify the etiologic factors for periodontal disease which will specify the possibility of tooth sustainability in short term and long term. Identification of individual tooth prognosis is an integral part of dental practice as it allows for an interdisciplinary approach in treatment strategies. Overall prognosis is advantageous for communication between patient and professionals.

The signs of active periodontal disease are bleeding on probing, pocket formation, suppuration and colour changes in gingiva. Without giving proper attention to it and not controlling the active periodontal inflammation, underlying periodontal disease may aggravate further leading to bone loss and loss of teeth. So, it is very important to eliminate active periodontal/peri implant disease prior to prosthetic constructions. In other words, long term prognosis of the prosthesis will be compromised if periodontal disease remain uncontrolled after delivery. Furthermore, untreated periodontal inflammation gives rise to soft tissue changes like colour, size, texture and consistency of gingiva which leads to impaired aesthetic outcome by collapsing the harmony between periodontium and prosthesis [38]. Periodontists play a significant role in managing hard and soft tissue around the prepared sites for successful and long term prosthesis. Bone augmentation, soft tissue augmentation, correction of existing ridge deformities and sinus lifting can be well handled by a periodontist for future implant sites.

Regular periodontal maintenance is a key to reduce the incidence of tooth or implant loss following prosthetic therapy.

2.6.3 The impact of prosthetic factors on periodontal/peri-implant health

Prosthodontist should properly design the prosthesis in consonance with the surrounding periodontium for long term maintenance of periodontal/peri implant health. Faulty restoration tends to accumulate plaque and food debris, thereby increasing periodontal disease progression. Violation of biologic width also result in periodontal inflammation.

2.6.4 Concept of biologic width and its applications in placement of margin

Understanding and clinically managing the concept of biological width is the key to creating gingival harmony with dental restoration. The dimension of dentogingival complex, called biological width is a cuff like barrier that acts as a protective physiological seal around natural teeth. It is defined as the dimension of space occupied by the soft tissues above the alveolar crest, so now the terminology of biological width is replaced by "Supracrestal attachment" in 2017 classification of periodontal disease. The connective tissue attachment occupied 1.07 mm above the level of the crestal bone, junctional epithelium attachment below the base of the gingival sulcus to be 0.97 mm. Encroachment on the biologic width by tooth preparation, caries, fracture, restorative materials or orthodontic devices can lead to bacterial accumulation, persistent gingival inflammation eventually resulting in increased probing depths, gingival recession or periodontal pocket formation [48].

2.6.5 Assessment of biologic width

Wilson and Maynard have described the concept of intra-crevicular restorative dentistry [49]. The restorative dentist must be able to determine the base of sulcus for intracrevicular margin location. Kois et al. suggested that the restorative dentist must be able to determine the total distance from the gingival crest to the alveoral crest. This procedure can be performed by bone sounding or transgingival probing. Based on the measurement during bone sounding three categories of biologic width can be described [50]:

1. Normal crest- Biologic width 3 mm, crown margin 0.5 mm subgingival.

2. High crest- Biologic width < 3 mm, does not allow subgingival margin placement without bone removal.

3. Low Crest-Biologic width > 3 mm, susceptible to recession if margin placed subgingivally.

2.6.6 Correction of violation of biologic width

To restore gingival health, it is necessary to re-establish the space clinically between alveolar bone and the gingival margin. For this either, surgery with or without bone alteration or orthodontic treatment to move the restorative margin away from bone level is done.

2.6.7 Margin placement guidelines

Rule-1: If the sulcus probes 1.5 mm or less, place to restoration margin 0.5 mm below the gingival tissue crest.

Rule 2: If the sulcus probes more than 1.5 mm, place the margin one half the depth of the sulcus below the tissue crest.

Rule-3: If the sulcus probes >2 mm especially on the facial aspect of the tooth, then evaluate to see whether gingivectomy could be performed to lengthen the crown and create a 1.5 mm sulcus. Then patient can be treated as mentioned in Rule-1 [51].

2.6.8 Current trends in periodontal aspects of restorative dentistry

- Supragingival placement of margins of restorations.

- Avoidance of over contoured restoration and minimal concern with lack of contour

- Occlusal stability through precise occlusal adjustment and accurate

- reconstruction of occlusal anatomy in single restorations.

- Restricted indication for splinting of mobile teeth.

- Hemisection with fixed bridges in cases of extensive furcation involvement.

2.6.9 Periodontal therapy before prosthodontic procedures

- A thorough periodontal evaluation is indicated on the planning stages prior to fabrication of the prosthesis. Selection of abutment teeth is based on prosthodontic and periodontal considerations, including bone support and architecture, width of attached gingiva, tooth mobility, root anatomy and tooth position.

- controlling or eliminating periodontal disease with cause related therapy and surgical therapy to eliminate pockets

- correction of gingival architecture that may favour disease, impair aesthetics or impede placement of prosthesis with preprosthetic surgery

- periodontal maintenance and motivation for oral hygiene should be given during treatment and interim periods.

An interdisciplinary approach requiring coordinated efforts by the Prosthodontist and Periodontist is the need of the hour. Close attention paid to both soft and hard tissues around teeth and implants before, during and after restorative procedure produces a successful outcome. It also gives the patient the benefit of comprehensive treatment with precise and long lasting restorations.

2.7 Interrelationship between endodontics and periodontics

The pulp periodontal interrelationship is a unique one and consider them as a single continuous system or as one biologic unit in which there are so many paths of communication [52]. The intricacy of endo-perio lesions (EPL) throws back the intimate relationship between the periodontal complex and endodontics [53].

The EPL terminology was first instituted in 1998 in the American association of endodontic, Glossary of endodontic terms. Later on American academy of Periodontology accepted this terminology and defined EPL to be localised infection beginning from pulpal or periodontal tissue [54]. Endo perio lesions are mostly anaerobic infections and polymicrobial in nature. The aetiology of EPL lesion is due to concurrent inflammation of variable magnitude of periodontal complex and endodontics. Causative factors are mostly bacterial origin. Dental malformations, history of trauma, iatrogenic perforations, external or internal root resorptions are also responsible for the endo-perio lesion. The existence of active tooth decay, furcation defect, anatomical grooves and porcelain fused to metal crowns are regarded as liability factors in the existence of EPL.

2.7.1 Pathways of EPL

There are several pathways of communication of infectious substances from pulp to periodontal tissue and vice versa. This in combination with the existing polymicrobial anaerobic infection leads to development of EPL [55].

The apical foramina and lateral canals link the pulpo-perio complex. Deep periodontal pocket reaching beyond the apical third of tooth can be connected to endodontic system through apical foramen. Lateral canals which are found all along the root surface give out a more accessible pathway for micro-organisms to travel from one tissue to other.

Any endodontic infection in the root apex can move up through periodontal ligament reaching the marginal gingiva and can increase periodontal disease severity by increasing pocket depth. This was termed as retrograde periodontitis [56]. Inversely microorganisms and noxious irritants can invade through dentinal tubules to the pulpal complex after the gradual loss of attached periodontal tissue.

1. There are certain treatment errors which can lead to combined EPL: Tooth decay on outer root surface beneath CEJ and improperly placed restoration

2. Root cracks resulting from high forces exerted during biomechanical preparation of rot canals.

3. Accidental perforation during endodontic treatment.

2.7.2 Classification system

Recent classification system of periodontal conditions, combined EPL are placed in the "periodontal manifestations of systemic diseases and developmental and acquired conditions" section and "other periodontal conditions" subsection.

Classification of EPLs modified from Simon et al.:

1. Primary endodontic lesions

2. Primary endodontic lesions with secondary periodontal involvement

3. Primary periodontal lesions

4. Primary periodontal lesions with secondary endodontic involvement

5. True combined lesions (**Table 1**)

DOI: http://dx.doi.org/10.5772/intechopen.99265

Tests	Primary endodontic lesion	Primary periodontal lesion	Primary endodontic secondary periodontal	Primary periodontal secondary endodontic	True Combined lesions
Visual	Presence of decay/incorrect restorations/ erosion/ abrasion	Inflammation /gingival recession Presence of plaque/ calculus Intact teeth	Plaque/ Calculus at the gingival margin Root perforation/ fracture	Plaque/ Calculus and swelling around multiple teeth Pus+Exudate	Periodontitis around single or multiple teeth Pus+Exudate
Pain	Sharp	Usually dull ache	Usually sharp	Usually dull ache	Usually dull ache,sharp only in acute condition
Palpation	Not conclusive	Pain on palpation	Pain on palpation	Pain on palpation	Pain on palpation
Percussion	Normally tender	Tender on percussion	Tender on percussion	Tender on percussion	Tender on percussion
Mobility	Present only in fractured or traumatised teeth	Localised/ generalised mobility	Localised mobility	Generalised mobility	Generalised higher grade mobility on involved tooth
Pulp vitality	Lingering or no response	Positive	Negative	Positive	Usually negative
Pocket probing	Solitary narrow pocket	Multiple wide and deep pockets	Solitary wide pockets	Multiple wide and deep pockets	Typical conic periodontal type of probing
Sinus tracing	Radiograph with gutta-percha points to apex/ furcation	At lateral aspect of the root	Mainly at the apex/ furcation	At lateral aspect of the root	Difficult to trace
X-rays	Periapical radiolucency	Vertical bone loss Wider bone loss	Wide based apical radiolucency	Angular bone loss in multiple teeth	Similar to a vertically fractured tooth
Cracked tooth Testing	Painful when chewing	No symptoms	Painful when chewing	No symptoms	Painful when chewing

Table 1.
Diagnostic examinations used to classify EPL adapted from Parolia et al. 2013 [57].

2.7.3 Treatment options

Correct diagnosis is key to management and prognosis of EPL. The most vital parameters to be considered while planning the treatment should be pulp vitality and extent of periodontal lesion. The prognosis of primary endodontic lesion is usually good if proper irrigation protocol is followed during cleaning and shaping and they heal with proper endodontic treatment [58].

Primary periodontal lesions can be treated by periodontal therapy only. Removing entire etiologic elements that can induce or promote epithelial down-growth followed by periodontal surgery is the best treatment modality in these cases [59].

True combined lesions are challenges that necessitate endodontic and periodontic regenerative treatment. As an initial step, true combined EPL should be treated endodontically first followed by other etiological factor management including periodontal management. If root resection or hemisection of molar teeth is planned, clinician must think of multiple factors like tooth restorability, regeneration of bone around sound root structure and concurrence of the patient. Prognosis of teeth can be ameliorated by osseous regeneration and Guided Tissue Regeneration (GTR). Endo-perio lesions are threat to dentists as multidisciplinary approach is required to acquire a positive result.

3. Conclusions

Interdisciplinary approach in periodontics includes a structured collaboration between periodontist and other specialists including allied health professionals involved in patient treatment. Furthermore, there is a common working knowledge between all. Now it is evidence based that Periodontics cannot be practised in isolation because for almost every case, there are multiple treatment plans that will provide both clinical predictability and patient satisfaction in achieving a higher level of success. In the field of Periodontics and Implantology, it is well understood that to manage the demand of rehabilitation of function and satisfying the patients aesthetic demand, the clinicians should practise interdisciplinary approach. Interdisciplinary approach develops a classic relationship within various specialities of dentistry that should go hand in hand for the complete well being of the patient. In day-to-day dental practice, clinical periodontal practice share an intimate and inseparable relationship with endodontics, orthodontics and prosthetic dentistry as well as other specialities in multiple aspects including treatment plan, procedure execution, outcome achievement and maintenance. All phases of clinical dentistry are intimately related to a common objective. The preservation and maintenance of the natural dentition in health is of prime importance in an integrated interdisciplinary approach to periodontal care.

Author details

Subash Chandra Raj*, Shaheda Tabassum, Annuroopa Mahapatra and Kaushik Patnaik
Department of Periodontics, SCB Dental College and Hospital, Cuttack, Odisha, India

*Address all correspondence to: drsubash007@gmail.com

References

[1] Karl M , Lyons & Ivano D. Periodontology 2000;74:7-10.

[2] Christina Doulkeridou, Ioannis Vouros, Anastasios Petridis, Zarkadi Athanasia-Eirini, Charis Theodoridis. Interdisciplinary Approach in Periodontology - A Mini-Review and A Report of Two Complex Cases. Dental Research and Oral Health 2020: 107-120.

[3] Allen T, B. S. Jagdish P, Sreelakshmi, krishnapriya, Razeena S, menees Anosca L,Interdisciplinary Periodontics: A Review. European Journal of Pharmaceutical and medical research 2019 research 2019;6: 230-237.

[4] Nancarrow SA, Booth A, Ariss S, Smith T, Enderby P, Roots A. Ten principles of good interdisciplinary team work. Hum Resour Health. 2013 10;11:19.

[5] Lancet T. oral health: prevention is key. Lancet 2009; 373:11-13.

[6] Chrisopoulos CB , Harbord JE. oral health and dental care in Australia:key facts and figures 2011. cat. No. DEN 224 Canberra AIHW, 2013.

[7] Scannapieco FA, Bush RB, Paju S. Associations between periodontal disease and risk for nosocomial bacterial pneumonia and chronic obstructive pulmonary disease. A systematic review. Ann Periodontol. 2003;8:54-69.

[8] Lopez JN, Uribe S, martinez B. Periodontal therapy reduces the rate of preterm low weight in women with Pregnancy associated gingivitis. J Periodontol 2005; 76:2144-2153.

[9] Nibali L, D'Aiuto F, Griffiths G, Patel K, Suvan J, Tonetti MS. Severe periodontitis is associated with systemic inflammation and a dysmetabolic status: a case-control study. J Clin Periodontol. 2007;34:931-7.

[10] Proussaefs P. Clinical and histologic evaluation of the use of mandibular tori as donor site for mandibular block autografts: A report of three cases. Int J Periodontics Restorative Dent 2006; 26: 43-51.

[11] Kim DH, Won SY, Choi DY, Kim HS, Jung UW, Kim HJ, Hu KS. Topography of the submental artery that should be considered in bleeding during dentoalveolar surgery. J Craniofac Surg. 2012 ;23:1453-6.

[12] Bernstein S, Cooke J, Fotek P, Wang HL. Vertical bone augmentation: where are we now? Implant Dent. 2006;15:219-28.

[13] American Academy of Paediatric Dentistry. Periodontal diseases of children and adolescents.Pediatr Dent 2014;35:338-345.

[14] FDI, A simplified Periodontal examination for dental practices based on the community Periodontal index of treatment needs – CPITN. Paris; FDI, 1986.

[15] Andreasen JO. Pulp and periodontal tissue repair - regeneration or tissue metaplasia after dental trauma. A review. Dent Traumatol. 2012; 28:19-24.

[16] Centers for disease control and prevention. youth and tobacco. use http:/www.cdc.gov/tobacco/data_statistics/fact_sheets/youth_data/tobacco_use/index.htm# estimates (Accessed 31st August 2014].

[17] Ayo-Yusuf OA, Reddy PS, van den Borne BW. Adolescents' sense of coherence and smoking as longitudinal predictors of self-reported gingivitis. J Clin Periodontol. 2008;35:931-7.

[18] Franchini R, Petri A, Migliario M, Rimondini L: Poor oral hygiene and gingivitis are associated with obesity

and overweight status in paediatric subjects. J Clin Periodontol 2011; 38: 1021-1028.

[19] Dyment HA, Casas MJ Dental care for children fed by tube: A critical review. Spec care Dent 1999;19:220-224.

[20] Jeevan M, Manjusha M, Gaurav H., ortho- perio synergy - A review, Mod Res Dent 2018; 1(4): 65-71 21.

[21] Suma Shekar, A. Bhagyalakshmi, B. R. Chandrasekhar, B.S. Avinash. Periodontal considerations during orthodontic treatment. Indian J Oral Health Res 2017;3:1-8.

[22] Shekar Suma & Lakshmi, Chandra shekar B R & Shivamallu Avinash. Periodontal considerations during orthodontic treatment. Indian Journal of Oral Health and Research. 2017;3:1-8.

[23] Vinod K, Reddy YG, Reddy VP, Nandan H, Sharma M. Orthodontic - Periodontic interdisciplinary approach. J Indian Soc Periodontal 2012; 16: 11-15.

[24] Aggarwal I, Tandon R, Srivastava S, Gupta. Ortho perio integration: An orthodontic review.Indian Journal of multidisciplinary Dentistry 2016;6: 99-103.

[25] Anna Marie R, Piotor SF, Alianne R, Rosemie K, Christos K. Am J Ortho Dentofacial orthop 2013;143:2016-12.

[26] Steiner GG, Pearson JK, Ainamo J. Changes of the marginal periodontium as a result of labial tooth movement in monkeys. J Periodontol. 1981 ;52:314-20.

[27] Greenbaum KR, Zachrisson BU. The effect of palatal expansion therapy on the periodontal supporting tissues. Am J Orthod. 1982 Jan;81(1):12-21. doi: 10.1016/0002-9416(82)90283-4. PMID: 6758588.

[28] Erkan M, Pikdoken L, Usumez S. Gingival response to mandibular incisor intrusion. Am J Orthod Dentofacial Orthop. 2007 Aug;132(2):143.e9-13. doi: 10.1016/j.ajodo.2006.10.015. PMID: 17693359.

[29] Jin L. Periodontic-orthodontic interactions rationale sequence and clinical implications. Hong kong Dent J 2007;4:60-64.

[30] Moyers RE, Dryland Vig KW, Fonseca R. Adult treatment.in: Moyers RE(Ed), Handbook of orthodontics (4th edn), Year book medical publisher inc, Chicago, USA, pp. 472-510.

[31] Mattingly JA, Sauer GJ Yancey JM, Arnold RR. Enhancement of Streptococcus mutans colonization by direct bonded orthodontic appliances. J Dent Res. 1983 ;62:1209-11.

[32] Paolantonio M, Festa F, di Placido G, D'Attilio M, Catamo G, Piccolomini R. Site-specific subgingival colonization by Actinobacillus actinomycetemcomitans in orthodontic patients. Am J Orthod Dentofacial Orthop. 1999;115:423-8.

[33] Deepa D, Mehta DS, Puri VK, Shetty S. Combined periodontic-orthodonticendodontic interdisciplinary approach in the treatment of periodontally compromised tooth. J Indian Soc Periodontol. 2010 Apr;14(2):139-43. doi: 10.4103/0972-124X.70837. PMID: 21691554; PMCID: PMC3110470.

[34] Vanarsadall RL. Periodontal Problems Associated with Orthodontic Treatment. The American Academy of Periodontics. 1981;3:154-157.

[35] Perinetti G, Paolantonio M, Serra E, D'Archivio D, D'Ercole S, Festa F, Spoto G. Longitudinal monitoring of subgingival colonization by Actinobacillus actinomycetemcomitans, and crevicular alkaline phosphatase and aspartate aminotransferase activities around orthodontically treated teeth. J Clin Periodontol. 2004;31:60-7.

[36] Devishree, & Gujjari, Sheela & Shubhashini, P.V. Frenectomy: A Review with the Reports of Surgical Techniques. Journal of clinical and diagnostic research: JCDR. 2012;6: 1587-92.

[37] Diedrich P. Periodontal relevance of anterior crowding. J Orofac Orthop. 2000;61:69-79.

[38] Yung-Ting,Nan-Chieh H, Hom –Lay W. The relationship between periodontics and prosthodontics: the two-way street. Journal of Prosthodontics and Implantology 2015;4:4-11.

[39] John P, Ambooken M, Kuriakose A, Mathew JJ. The perio-restorative interrelationship-expanding the horizons in esthetic dentistry. J Interdiscip Dentistry 2015;5:46-53.

[40] Becker CM, Kaldahi WB. Current theories of crown contour, margin placement, and pontic design.J Prosthet Dent 1981;45:268-77.

[41] Schlugers, Yuodells RA, Page RC. Periodontal disease. Philadelphia:Lea and febiger 1977:586-617.

[42] Kois JC. The restorative-periodontal interface: biological parameters. Periodontol 2000. 1996;11:29-38.

[43] Vacaru, R., Podariu, A., Jumanca, D., Găluşcan, A., & Muntean, R. Periodontal-restorative interrelationships. oral health Dent Med Bas Sci 2003;3:12-5.

[44] Eissmann HF, Radke RA, Noble WH. Physiologic design criteria for fixed dental restorations. Dent Clin North Am. 1971 ;15:543-68.

[45] Goldberg PV, Higginbottom FL, Wilson TG. Periodontal considerations in restorative and implant therapy. Periodontol 2000. 2001;25:100-9.

[46] Morris ML. Artificial crown contours and gingival health. J Prosthet Dent 1962;12:11-46.

[47] Stein RS. Pontic-residual ridge relationship: a research report. J Prosthet Dent. 1966 Mar-Apr;16(2):251-85. doi: 10.1016/0022-3913(66)90080-1. PMID: 5217111.

[48] Tal H, Soldinger M, Dreiangel A, Pitaru S. Periodontal response to long-term abuse of the gingival attachment by supracrestal amalgam restorations. J Clin Periodontol. 1989;16:654-9.

[49] Wilson RD, Maynard G. Intracrevicular restorative dentistry. Int J Periodontics Restorative Dent. 1981;1-35.

[50] Robbins JW.Tissue Management in Restorative Dentistry Functional Esthetics & Restor Dent 2007;1:40-3.

[51] Melnick, Philip.Preparation of the Periodontium for Restorative Dentistry. in: Carrana's clinical periodontology.10th edition Philadelphia:WB Saunders co:2003.825-831.

[52] Parolia A, Gait TC, Porto IC, Mala K. Endo-perio lesion: A dilemma from 19 th until 21 st century. J Interdiscip Dentistry 2013;3:2-11.

[53] Dakó, Timea & Lazăr, Ana & Bică, Cristina & Lazar, Luminita. Endo-perio lesions: diagnosis and interdisciplinary treatment options. Acta Stomatologica Marisiensis Journal2020;3:257-261.

[54] Shenoy N, Shenoy A. Endo-perio lesions: diagnosis and clinical considerations. Indian J Dent Res. 2010;21:579-85.

[55] Zehnder M, Gold SI, Hasselgren G. Pathologic interactions in pulpal and periodontal tissues. J Clin Periodontol. ; 29:663-71.

[56] Rotstein I, Simon JH. Diagnosis, prognosis and decision-making in the treatment of combined periodontal-endodontic lesions. Periodontol 2000. 2004;34:165-203.

[57] Parolia A, Gait TC, Porto IC, Mala K. Endo-perio lesion: A dilemma from 19 th until 21 st century. J Interdiscip Dentistry 2013;3:2-11.

[58] Carrotte P. Endodontics: Part 9. Calcium hydroxide, root resorption, endo-perio lesions. Br Dent J. 2004;197:735-43.

[59] Miao H, Chen M, Otgonbayan T et al. Papillary reconstruction and guided tissue regeneration for combined periodontal–endodontic lesions caused by palatogingival groove and additional root: a case report 2015;3:1042-49.

Chapter 4

Orthodontic-Periodontics: An Interdisciplinary Approach

Shreya Kishore, Vanita Barai, Suvetha Siva and Keerthi Venkatesan

Abstract

Periodontal pathogenesis is a multi-factorial process and the orthodontist must recognize the clinical forms of inflammatory periodontal disease. Orthodontics is the most conservative and predictable treatment to improve numerous local etiological factors that contribute to periodontal disease including periodontal breakdown. Proper occlusal function and masticatory function are stimulatory to the gingival tissue and the attachment apparatus, while, conversely, a lack of function predisposes to disease that increases plaque retention and calculus formation along with gingival inflammation leading to increased loss of bony support. No matter how talented the orthodontist, a magnificent orthodontic correction can be destroyed by failure to recognize periodontal susceptibility. Therefore, identifying periodontally susceptible patients is critical for the outcome of the treatment. This chapter will highlight the importance of the short-term and long-term outcomes of orthodontic treatment, which are influenced by the patient's periodontal status before, during and after active orthodontic therapy.

Keywords: Bio-relationship, Interdisciplinary approach, Adjunctive periodontal procedures, Periodontium, Orthodontia, Periodontal healing

1. Introduction

Periodontal care should be directed towards eliminating the bacterial infection and preventing reinfection. This involves creating an environment which encourages self-cleansing and is less conducive to harboring pathogenic bacteria. Appropriate therapy for each individual depends on the type, severity and morphology created by the specific disease, along with cooperation from the patient. Regardless, elimination of as many plaque-retentive areas should always be the primary objective of a treatment. Large number of teeth are extracted to eliminate periodontal defects (that act as bacterial reservoirs) that can be corrected by simple tooth eruption [1].

Although orthodontic treatment may not be considered preventive or corrective of periodontitis, it is one of the solutions to reduce the local factors. Patients with predisposing periodontal health tend to experience movement in teeth, as there will be comparatively lesser periodontal support. Commonly occurring movements of teeth include migration of teeth, intrusion, extrusion and flaring of teeth. In such cases, orthodontic treatment helps in eliminating the malposition of teeth but also aids in long term maintenance [2].

2. Role of periodontics in orthodontic treatment

When moving teeth orthodontically, the entire periodontal attachment apparatus, including the osseous structure, the PDL, and the soft tissue components, move with the tooth. Even though the connective tissue attachment level remains unchanged along the root surface there are considerable morphological alterations to crestal bone with tooth uprighting [3]. Hence we can say that orthodontic treatment is almost always an interdisciplinary approach, where the health of the periodontium plays a vital role throughout the treatment. Certain techniques can be adjunctive to the Orthodontic treatment which will be discussed further in this chapter.

2.1 Soft tissue considerations

2.1.1 Adjunctive procedures

They can majorly be classified, based on the extent and involvement, as, minimal, moderate and severe involvement. The procedures are discussed in the following.

2.1.1.1 Minimal involvement

2.1.1.1.1 Fiberotomy

Also known as circumferential supracrestal fiberotomy (CSF), it is one of the common procedures conducted to enhance retention after fixed orthodontic therapy. The procedure involves detachment of the supracrestal fibers to increase the retention of a re-established tooth position. Tooth repositioning (for e.g.: rotation) is tough in maintenance. To accommodate the new tooth position after orthodontic therapy, reorganization of the PDL fibers take place. This rearrangement of fibers, especially the Sharpe's fibers, take place even after 6 months, due to which the retention period is always advised for a minimum of 12 months [4].

Literature suggests that the maximum amount of relapse takes place during the first 5 hours post the removal of the appliance. Hence it is ideal for fiberotomy to be done at the end of the finishing phase of orthodontic therapy. This minimizes the relapse that usually occurs due to the elastic supracrestal gingival fibers [3].

2.1.1.1.2 Frenectomy

A frenectomy is a procedure that removes the frenum (a small muscular attachment that connects two pieces of oral tissue) (**Figures 1** and **2**). Labial frenum is present apical, between the two central incisors. Most commonly, the maxillary labial frenum tends to be more muscular causing midline diastema. In such cases apart from orthodontic therapy, adjuvant frenectomy procedure aids in space closure ensuring lesser chances of relapse. Usually the surgical removal of frenum is done after orthodontic treatment is complete or during the finishing phase of active orthodontic treatment [5].

2.1.1.1.3 Gingivectomy and gingivoplasty

Gingivectomy is a dental procedure, where a part of the gingiva is surgically removed (**Figures 3** and **4**). It is an essential and adjunctive procedure to orthodontic therapy. Gingivoplasty, on the other hand, is the reshaping of the gingiva

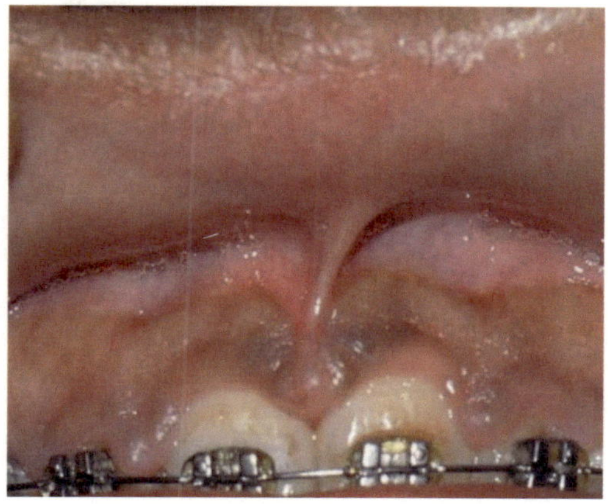

Figure 1.
High labial frenum (pre-operative).

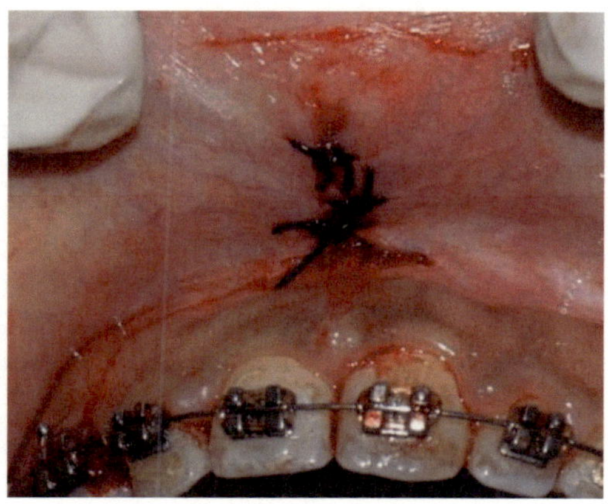

Figure 2.
Post-operative picture of Frenectomy.

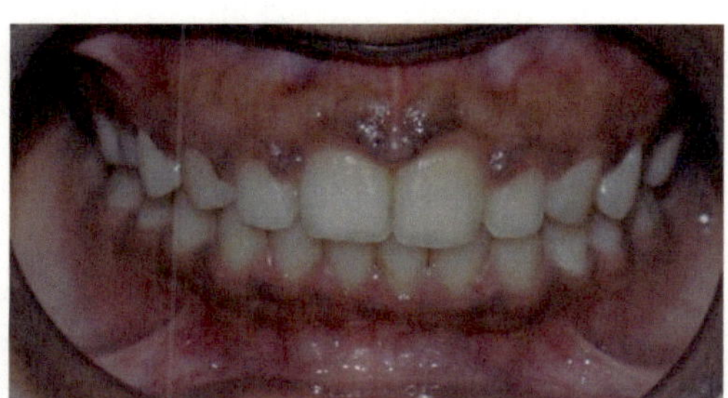

Figure 3.
Uneven gingival margins (pre–operative).

to re-create physiologic contours with the purpose of recontouring the gingiva in the absence of pockets. Gingivectomy and gingivoplasty procedures are commonly performed together [6]. They are usually done for improving esthetics and for enhancing the prognosis of the teeth. Gingivectomy is needed in areas of space closure, where the tissue bunching also called clefts are surgically removed. It has also been documented that, performing CSF during a forced eruption of a tooth prevents displacement of gingiva more coronally [7, 8]. This will reduce the requirement for gingival recontouring after the completion of tooth movement.

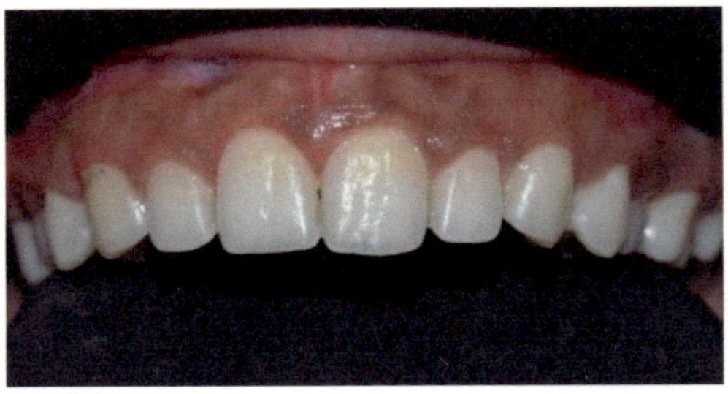

Figure 4.
Post-operative picture gingivectomy done to correct the uneven margins.

2.1.1.2 Moderate involvement

2.1.1.2.1 Depigmentation

Gingival hyperpigmentation is presented as a diffuse, deep purplish, discoloration or irregularly shaped brown, light brown or black patches, striae or strands seen in the attached gingiva. This may be a genetic trait in some populations and is more appropriately termed as a physiologic or racial gingival pigmentation. This is common in occurrence and is immensely disturbing to the esthetics, especially while smiling [7, 8].

Gingival hyperpigmentation may be caused by exogenous and endogenous factors. Exogenous factors include contact with heavy metals and smoking. Endogenous factors include endocrine and genetic disorders. Clinical hyperpigmentation of the gingiva does not necessarily present as a medical problem. Gingival depigmentation is a periodontal procedure, to restore a more natural color of the mucosa [8].

2.1.1.2.2 Guided tissue regeneration

The aim of regenerative therapy is the restoration of lost tissue in its form and function. GTR is a surgical procedure that uses barrier membranes to direct the growth of new bone and gingival tissue to sites with insufficient volume or dimension of bone and gingiva for proper function, esthetics and prosthetic rehabilitation [9]. GTR is used as an adjunct to orthodontics to re-establish new periodontal attachment and to improve the pre-orthodontic conditions for moving the teeth into infrabony defects or for guiding vertical movements of teeth with reduced bone support [10].

2.1.1.2.3 Gingival curettage

Gingival curettage is a surgical procedure designed to remove the infected/ affected soft tissue lining of the periodontal pocket with a curet, leaving only a gingival connective tissue lining (**Figures 5** and **6**). The purpose of curettage is to eliminate or reduce the depth of the periodontal pocket by promoting the shrinkage of gingiva and enhancing new connective tissue attachment [11].

1. In cases of the presence of mild to moderate pockets, gingival curettage can be done to improve gingival attachments.

2. In cases where aggressive treatment is contraindicated, it can be performed to reduce the gingival inflammation.

3. In cases of recurrent inflammation, gingival curettage can be done to maintain gingival health.

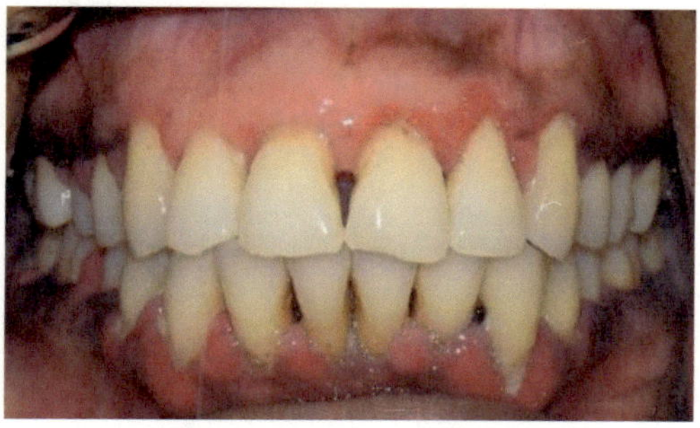

Figure 5.
Pre-operative picture, presence of deep pockets.

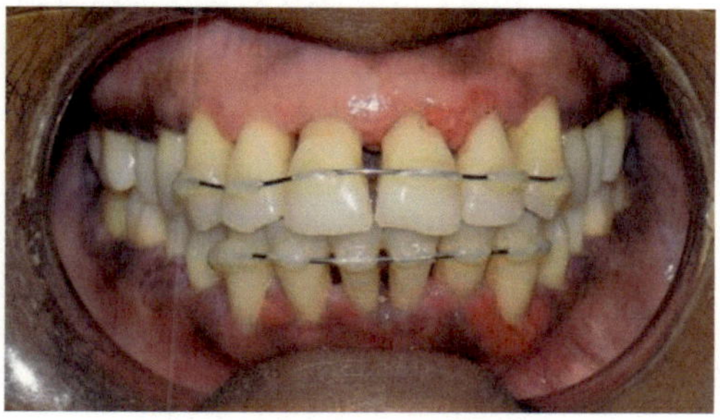

Figure 6.
Post-operative–full mouth curettage done.

In many cases, it may be possible to correct bony pockets by correcting the tooth position and allowing reestablishment of the periodontal apparatus with the help of orthodontics [12]. A combination of orthodontics and periodontal therapy may help to improve the periodontal status and maintenance of oral health for a patient [13].

2.1.1.2.4 Crown lengthening

Crown lengthening is usually done to correct a gummy smile or fix a clinically short crown height for a tooth that requires bonding or banding.

When malalignment is responsible for a gummy smile, a gingival surgery is not the first treatment of choice, the teeth, then must be moved to a more esthetic and functional position, and the smile is corrected by an orthodontic leveling of the gingival margins.

It's important for the periodontist and orthodontist to identify the cases in which the teeth can be treated by gingival surgery and the ones in which orthodontics can benefit [12–14].

A gummy smile, may occur due to 3 reasons, the first being a maxillary excess, which is usually treated with a combination of orthodontics and surgery [14], secondly, a short anatomic lip and thirdly, the excessive eruption of maxillary teeth with delayed apical migration over the maxillary anterior can cause a gummy smile.

For gingivectomy or crown lengthening the sulcular depth is 3-4 mm when it should be only 1 mm, it may not migrate easily towards the CEJ, hence it has to be corrected [15].

Gingival margin discrepancy can be assessed by 4 parameters

1. Relation between the gingival margin of the maxillary central incisor and the patients lip line

2. Evaluate the labial sulcular depth

3. Evaluate the relation between the shortest central incisor and the adjacent lateral incisor.

4. Assess the incisal edges for abrasion

In some cases, the molars may have a short crown height and the placement of an orthodontic band can lead to attachment loss due to the encroachment of the biologic width. To prevent these problems, a crown lengthening procedure should be considered prior to the placement of orthodontic bands used for anchorage.

To achieve the appropriate crown to root ratio for orthodontic bonding, one may need to do a crown lengthening procedure [16] as this is a crucial step and can aid in a more specific outcome in treatment planning.

2.1.1.2.5 Gingival recession and root coverage

Gingival recession is not due to Orthodontics, it may be a multifactorial issue (**Figures** 7 and **8**) [17]. There are many ways to cover a recession, and various grafting techniques are available [18]. Conventionally, gingival and pedicle grafts were used for root coverage previously, but presently connective tissue grafts are the treatment of choice to cover root exposures [19]. The advantages are, greater root coverage, superior esthetics and the ease and patient comfort.

Usually, the grafting is conducted after the completion of orthodontic treatment, however in many circumstances, due to inadequate gingiva and detrimental recession, the procedure may be done before or during Orthodontic treatment. This is usually case specific.

The factors to be considered before deciding for intervention.

1. Esthetics.

2. Sensitivity.

3. Depth of root erosion.

4. Patients concerns regarding the treatment.

5. Any gingival restorations.

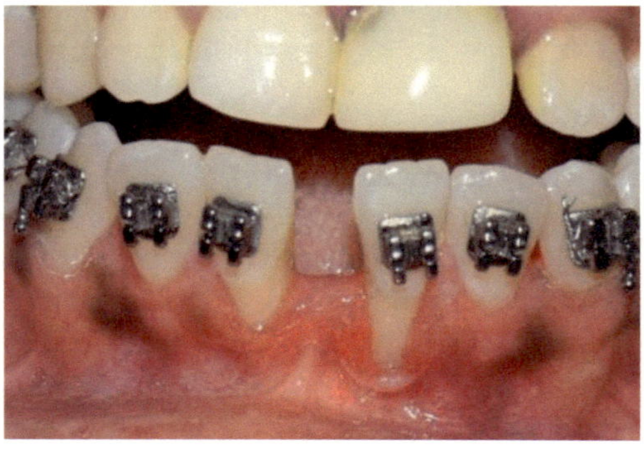

Figure 7.
Pre–operative: gingival recession in relation to 31.

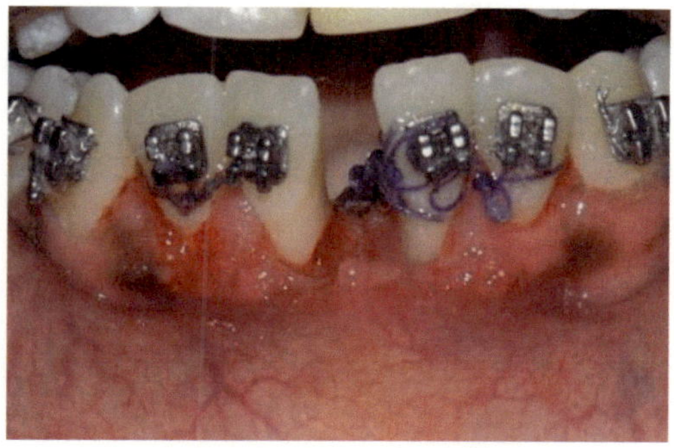

Figure 8.
Post-operative: root coverage done in relation to 31.

2.1.1.3 Severe involvement

2.1.1.3.1 Corticotomy

Corticotomy – it is a minor surgical procedure defined as osteotomy of cortical bone (**Figure 9**) [20]. Since the primary resistance to tooth movement is encountered in the cortical layer, corticotomy procedure makes it possible to move teeth faster without undesirable side effects [21].

How can corticotomy be used along with Orthodontics?

1. Exposure of impacted teeth by corticotomy assissted orthodontics

2. Intrusion of overerupted molars by corticotomy.

3. Rapid retraction of severely proclined incisors with spacing

4. Closure of fistula by bony transport and corticotomy assissted expansion.

5. In cases with significant arch-length discrepancies.

6. In cases with transversely constricted maxilla.

7. To enhance molar distalization.

8. Corticotomy and compression osteogenesis in the posterior maxilla for treating severe anterior openbite

Suya suggested that most surgical and orthodontic procedures be performed in the first 3-4 months after corticotomy, before fusion of tooth bone units [22].

It is critical to begin the orthodontic movement immediately after the surgery, before bony healing occurs. Since it takes around 4 hours for the release of cAMP and as well as for bone remodeling to start; it will be better for us to activate the orthodontic phase of treatment immediately after the corticotomy procedure [23].

Frost coined the term, 'Regional Accelerated Phenomenon' (RAP), where he noticed that surgical healing occurred mainly at the surgical site due to the reorganization of cells and accelerated bone turnover rate.

The technique developed by the Wilckos, called the Wilckodontics system or Accelerated Osteogenic Orthodontics (AOO), is similar to single tooth corticotomy,

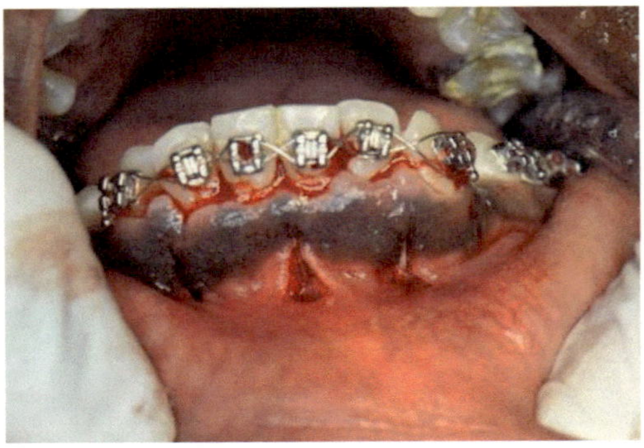

Figure 9.
Corticotomy done in the lower anterior region to induce the AOO phenomenon.

except that it is extended to all the teeth to be moved during orthodontic treatment (**Figure 1**). This usually aids with correction of severe malocclusions and crowding.

2.1.1.3.2 Bone grafts

Pre-orthodontic Osseous surgeries.

Osseous craters - these do not repair or improve with orthodontic treatment hence they should be treated before any orthodontics is initiated [23]. They are inter proximal two walled defects which may be maintainable non-surgically, however if correction or intervention is required then it can be managed with shaping the defect and reducing the pocket depth. The need for surgery is based on many factors like patient compliance, location of the defect, resistance to treatment by the periodontium [24].

3 walled defects- these usually require auto generous bone grafts or allografts with resorbable membranes [25]. If the results of periodontal therapy are stable post 3-6 months after, then orthodontic treatment maybe considered.

Types of bone grafts used.

1. Autografts

2. Allografts

3. Xenografts

4. Alloplastic

5. Non bone grafts

Bone grafting is very commonly done at many stages for cleft patients as an adjunct to the orthodontic treatment planning [26]. It has even been found that the canines organically are guided into the graft site also [27]. Hence grafting has been very essential part of orthodontics especially for cleft palate patients [28, 29].

Also it aids during cortication procedures. Many times to aid in tooth movements and to prevent the onset of any Osseous defects cortication is carried with a bone graft and the results are usually sound periodontium and excellent tooth movements. In many cases it also allows regeneration and restoration of the periodontium. With the help of a graft many difficult tooth movements can be continued in an otherwise compromised periodontium [30].

DOI: http://dx.doi.org/10.5772/intechopen.98627

3. Role of orthodontics in periodontal treatment

The patients who seek orthodontic treatment beyond the age of 18 are categorized as: (a) young adults (typically younger than 35 years, often in their 20s) who have not received any comprehensive orthodontic treatment in their teens and (b) an older group, typically in their 40s or 50s, who need orthodontics as a corrective measure for an interdisciplinary approach [13].

The first group often seek treatment to improve their quality of life. Their expectations are more and they seek the best possible outcome. While the latter need treatment, to improve and maintain their current oral health, not necessarily seeking treatment to achieve an esthetic outcome, hence correction and control of disease progression becomes the primary goal in this group of patients.

In adults, Adjunctive orthodontic treatment is, tooth movements that are planned and achieved to facilitate other dental procedures necessary to control disease, restore function, and/or enhance appearance. The primary goal is to make it easier or more effective to replace missing or damaged teeth and to control periodontal problems. The treatment duration tends to be a few months, rarely more than a year, and long-term retention often is supplied by the restorations. The treatment duration tends to be a few months, rarely more than a year, and long-term retention is provided with restorations.

3.1 Orthodontic considerations

Orthodontic therapy can provide various benefits to the periodontal patient as discussed here [11]:

- The malaligned maxillary or mandibular anterior teeth pose a challenge in maintaining a good oral hygiene.
- Patients with fractured maxillary anteriors can benefit with orthodontic treatment, where extrusion of the tooth can improve the crown and root ratio, as well as improve the quality of restoration provided to the tooth.
- Vertical repositioning of teeth by orthodontic forces can improve certain types of osseous defects in periodontal patients, minimizing or eliminating the need for resective osseous surgery.
- Orthodontic treatment can improve the esthetic relationship of gingival margin levels.
- Orthodontic treatment can help in improving the adjacent teeth position before the restorative phase.

3.1.1 Adjunctive procedures

3.1.1.1 Orthodontic treatment for osseous defects

According to the literature, there are three risk groups in a population for progression of periodontal bone loss: (a) those with rapid progression (about 10%), (b) those with moderate progression (the majority, about 80%), and (c) those with no progression (about 10%) [13, 30].

Patients who have had a history with periodontal disease and bone loss, present with no contraindication to receiving orthodontic treatment if the disease has been treated and maintained adequately since. The Periodontist usually guides the Orthodontist in this regard as progression of an untreated periodontal breakdown must be anticipated, however, the patient's periodontal condition must receive attention during planning and execution of orthodontic treatment [30].

3.1.1.2 Hemiseptal defects

Hemiseptal defects are one-or two-wall osseous defects that are often seen around mesially tipped teeth or supra-erupted teeth. Usually, these defects can be eliminated with orthodontic treatment [30, 31].

Some patients have a discrepancy between both the marginal ridges and the bone levels but these discrepancies may not be of equal magnitude; orthodontic leveling of the bone in this case may not be able to level the marginal ridges. In these patients the crowns of the teeth should not be used as a guide for completing orthodontic therapy. The bone should be leveled, and any remaining discrepancies between the marginal ridges should be equilibrated. In case of a tooth that is tipped, uprighting it will level the defect [31].

If there is supraeruption, then, intrusion and leveling the tooth, can help in leveling the osseous defect. It is important that any periodontal inflammation be controlled before the start of orthodontic therapy. After the completion of orthodontic treatment, these teeth should be stabilized for at least 6 months and reassessed periodontally.

3.1.1.3 Advanced horizontal bone loss

The location of the bands and brackets on the teeth is a primary determinant of outcome after orthodontic treatment has been planned. In a periodontally healthy individual, the anatomy of the crowns of the teeth determines the position of the brackets. Incisal edges and marginal ridges form a guide to position the anterior brackets and posterior bands or brackets. If the incisal edges and marginal ridges are at the correct level, the cementoenamel junction (CEJ) will also be at the same level. This relationship creates a flat, bony contour between the teeth [13, 32].

In situations where the patient has an underlying periodontal problems and significant alveolar bone loss around certain teeth, using the anatomy of the crown to determine bracket placement is not appropriate. In vital teeth, the equilibration should be performed gradually to allow the pulp to form secondary dentin and insulate the tooth during the equilibration process [32].

The main goal of equilibration and favorable bracket placement is to provide a constructive bony level as well as a more favorable crown-to-root ratio. In some of these patients, the initially apparent periodontal defects may not need periodontal surgery after orthodontic therapy.

3.1.1.4 Furcation defects

Furcation is the place where the roots of teeth separate. Furcation defect is bone loss, commonly due to a result of periodontal disease affecting the base of the root trunk of a tooth. These furcation defects can be classified as: Class I, Class II and Class III (mild, moderate and severe respectively) [11]. Furcation lesions require special consideration because they are difficult to maintain and can worsen during orthodontic therapy. These patients ideally should be on a 2 to 3 month recall schedule. Detailed instrumentation of the furcation can help minimize further periodontal breakdown.

The treatment modalities in a furcation defect usually involve hemisection (mostly in class III defects). After hemisection, and completion of endodontic and periodontal surgery, can the tooth serve as an abutment. Some molars with class III furcation defects, may have short roots, advanced bone loss, fused roots, or other conditions that contraindicate hemisection. In these patients, extraction and replacement with an implant is advisable [33] at any point irrespective, to the orthodontic treatment.

3.1.1.5 Root proximity

When roots of the posterior teeth are in proximity, periodontal health and restorative options are limited. With the help of orthodontics, these roots can be separated allowing bone to form, which widen the embrasures, provide additional bone support, and make oral hygiene more accessible. The movements should be planned prior to bonding, so they can progress with the initial arch wires. The movements can be monitored with radiographs. A movement of 2-3 mm is usually sufficient for favorable bone response. The oral hygiene maintenance should be good. Occasional occlusal adjustments may be required in the process [31, 33].

3.1.2 Fractured teeth and forced eruption

Trauma to the upper anterior is the most common occurrence in children and adolescents. This trauma can be (a) fracture of the crown or (b) fracture of crown and root. If the fracture is restricted to the crown, then endodontics and restorative procedures will be sufficient to manage. If the fracture extends into the biological width, then any restoration will cause irritation and inflammation to the marginal gingiva. Alternatively, extrusion of the tooth followed by restoration may be possible depending on the amount of tooth structure [34]. If the fracture extends to the root, then, depending on the level of involvement the tooth may have to be extracted. There are six criterias used to determine the direction of treatment to choose:

a. Root length: The ideal crown to root ratio should be 1:1 after extrusion of the tooth. In order to maintain the biological width of 2.5 mm, 4 mm should be extruded, this will provide 1.5 mm margin in crown preparation. The root length is evaluated using periapical radiographs. If this ratio is less than 1:1, the tooth will be unstable within the bone, hence extraction will be mandated.

b. Root form: Both the external and internal root form should be considered. The external root form should be broad and non-tapering rather than thin and tapering. This root form avoids easy fracture and unaesthetic appearance at the cervical margins after restoration. Internally, the root canal should be one-third of the root form in order to avoid root fracture.

c. Level of fracture: If the fracture level is 2-3 mm apical to the alveolar bone, the ideal treatment of choice will be extraction.

d. Age of the patient: If it is a young patient, forced eruption followed by the crown placement will be the ideal choice of treatment. If it is an aged patient with a crown on an adjacent tooth, it will be better to extract and replace the teeth.

e. Esthetics: If the patient has a high lip line, gingival exposure on smile will be increased. Hence, preservation of natural teeth will be better than artificial restoration of teeth.

f. Prognosis: Endodontically, if there are vertical fractures of the root, it should be extracted. Periodontally, if there is an osseous defect, then the tooth can be extracted [13, 32, 34].

If all the above criteria are favorable, forced eruption of teeth can be considered. It can be carried out with orthodontic brackets or with composite extension with elastics. If the tooth movement is faster, the bone will not follow the root, hence circumferential fibrotomy would be necessary. If the tooth movement is slow, the bone follows the root and crown lengthening procedure may be required for the restorative phase.

After the forced extrusion, teeth must be stabilized to prevent re-intrusion, which may occur due to the orientation of the oblique fibers, which will allow intrusion with any compressive force, until 6 months post treatment [33].

Usually during forced eruption, the clinical crown length may be shortened. This is because the gingiva follows the direction of eruption of the teeth. If there is a mismatch in the bone levels with the adjacent teeth, flap elevation and bone recontouring followed by gingivectomy can be considered. If the mismatch is limited only to the gingival heights then gingivectomy is sufficient [32, 34].

Post gingival surgery, embrasures due to the difference in the widths of root and crown may be seen. These can be corrected either by re- contouring the teeth or by reshaping the crowns during space closure. The latter is preferred because it improves the overall shape of the final crown [35].

3.1.2.1 Hopeless teeth maintained for orthodontic anchorage

In certain cases, moderate to severe periodontally compromised teeth may be used for anchorage. Even though the tooth is compromised, with sufficient bone it may be used for anchorage. Flap surgery and root debridement can improve the quality of this anchorage unit and post orthodontics, these can be maintained as are or extracted and replaced [36].

3.1.3 Orthodontic treatment of gingival discrepancies

3.1.3.1 Uneven gingival margins

The gingival margins of the anterior teeth play an important role in esthetics. The four factors that need to be considered for good esthetics are: (a) The height of the gingival margins of upper central incisors should be equal, (b) Gingival margin of lateral incisor should be coronal to the central incisor, (c) The gingival contour should follow the shape of CEJs in the anterior region, (d) Gingival papilla should occupy half the distance from the highest point of gingival contour to the incisal edge; the remaining half should be tooth contact [37].

The cause of the marginal discrepancies should be appropriately diagnosed and treated by either orthodontics or gingival surgery.

Four steps that can be considered for planning the treatment are: [36, 37]

Lip line: When the patient smiles, if the gingival discrepancy is not visible, it can be left untreated. If it is visible, then step two should be evaluated.

Labial sulcular depth: in the presence of an uneven gingival margin, if the labial sulcular depth is greater than 1 mm, then gingivectomy is possible. If the labial sulcular depth is less than 1 mm, then step three should be evaluated.

Relationship to the adjacent incisors: If the Central incisor is longer than the adjacent lateral incisor, orthodontic extrusion of this incisor will allow the gingival margins to move apically. The extruded tooth will have to be leveled with the adjacent teeth. If the Central incisor is shorter than the adjacent lateral incisor, then step four should be evaluated.

Abrasion: The incisal edges should be checked in the occlusal view. If this is thicker than the adjacent central incisor, then extrusion has taken place. Then the treatment of choice would be intrusion of the affected central incisors which will move the gingival margin apically. Followed by restoration of incisal edges. This step should be completed 6 months prior to the appliance removal as the periodontal fibers need time for re-orientation.

3.1.3.2 Significant abrasion and over eruption

When the patient reports with an abraded anterior, it can be managed either by orthodontic extrusion and restoration of the anterior tooth or by orthodontic intrusion of the adjacent anterior teeth followed by restoration of incisal edges. The extrusion option is not preferred as it may alter the crown: root ratio (1:1). It is advisable to intrude the anteriors. Extrusion of posterior teeth is not possible due to the occlusal forces. Once the intrusion has been achieved it is followed by a retention phase for 6 months after which restorations on the incisal edges can reestablish the ideal crown height [38].

3.1.3.3 Open gingival embrassures

The gingival embrasures can be deficit or open due to several reasons such as: (1) root position, (2) underlying bone loss, and (3) shape of the crown. If the problem is due to divergent roots, then orthodontic correction with modification of bracket position is an option. Once the root position is corrected, changes in the incisal contact can be modified. If the open gingival embrasure is due to other reasons, intrusion of the teeth would be ideal. Orthodontic intrusion will lead to compression of spaces which will in turn lead to an occlusal push of interdental gingiva, thus achieving the ideal ratio of 1:1, embrasure to tooth contact [34].

4. Conclusion

Adjunctive orthodontic treatment for patients with periodontal disease has some unique effects. Orthodontic treatment should only be done on a clinically sound periodontium. It is essential for dentists to have adequate knowledge on perio-ortho interrelationship. Maintaining a good oral hygiene and receiving regular basic periodontal care is of outmost importance to achieve a more effective orthodontic treatment. A better outcome can be achieved along with good maintenance, through a close collaboration between the orthodontist and the periodontist.

Acknowledgements

We would like to acknowledge the contribution of Dr. Kavarathapu Avinash, Periodontist and Implantologist, and Dr. Joseph Abraham, Orthodontist for generously sharing their clinical case photographs for our chapter.

Last but not the least, we would like to thank our parents and families, our teachers and mentors for their never-ending support and guidance.

Conflict of interest

The authors declare no conflict of interest.

Author details

Shreya Kishore[1*], Vanita Barai[2], Suvetha Siva[1] and Keerthi Venkatesan[3]

1 Faculty Orthodontist, SRM Dental College, Chennai, India

2 Orthodontic Consultant and Cosmetic Dentist, Calcutta, India

3 Faculty Orthodontist, SRIHER (DU), Chennai, India

*Address all correspondence to: dr.shreyakishore@gmail.com

References

[1] ROBERT L VANARSDALL. Orthodontics and periodontal therapy. Periodontol 2000. 1995;9:132-9.

[2] Brown LJ, Garci R. Utilization of dental servoces as a risl factor for periodontitis. J Periodontal. 1994;65: 551-63.

[3] Marianne M. A. Ong, Hom-Lay Wang. Periodontic and orthodontic treatment in adults. Am J Orthod Dentofac Orthop. 2002;(122):420-8.

[4] KAARE REITAN,. TISSUE BEHAVIOR DURING ORTHODONTIC TOOTH MOVEMENT. Am J Orthod. 1960 Dec;46(12):881-900.

[5] Jin L. Periodontic-orthodontic interactions—rationale, sequence and clinical implications. Hong Kong Dent J. 2007;4(1):60-4.

[6] Saroch N. Periobasics - A textbook of Periodontics and Implantology. 2nd ed. Sushrut Publications;

[7] Kozlovsky A, Tal H, Lieberman M. Forced eruption combined with gingival fiberotomy. J Clin Periodontol. 1988;15:534-8.

[8] Yenniy Ismullah, Shafira Kurnia. GINGIVECTOMY AND GINGIVAL DEPIGMENTASION AFTER ORTHODONTIC TREATMENT. DENTINO J Kedokt GIGI. 2020 Sep;5(2).

[9] Peter R. Diedrich. Guided Tissue Regeneration Associated With Orthodontic Therapy. Semin Orthod. 1996 Mar;2:39-45.

[10] Christoph Reichert, James Deschner, Adrian Kasaj, Andreas Jäger. Guided Tissue Regeneration and Orthodontics. A Review of the Literature. J Orofac Orthop. 2009;70:6-19.

[11] Newman, Takei, Klokkevold, Carranza. Carranza's Clinical Peridontology. 10th ed. Elsevier;

[12] Niklaus P Lang, Jan Lindhe. Clinical Periodontology and Implant Dentistry. 6th Edition. Vol. 1. Wiley Blackwell;

[13] William R Proffit, Raymond R White, David M Sarver. Contemporary Treatment of Dentofacial Deformity. Mosby Elseiver;

[14] K Willmar. On Le Fort I osteotomy; A follow-up study of 106 operated patients with maxillo-facial deformity. Scand J Plast Reconstr Surg. 1974;12.

[15] J G Maynard Jr, R D Wilson. Physiologic dimensions of the periodontium significant to the restorative dentist. J Periodontol. 1979;50(4).

[16] Vincent G. Kokich. Esthetics: the orthodontic-periodontic restorative connection. Semin Orthod [Internet]. 1996;2(1). Available from: https://doi.org/10.1016/S1073-8746(96)80036-3

[17] Mathews, Vincent K. Interdisciplianry Treatment: Integrating orthodontics with Periodontics, Endodontics and Restorative Dentistry. Semin Orthod. 1997 Mar;3(1).

[18] PRESTON D. MILLER JR, EDWARD P. ALLEN. The development of periodontal plastic surgery. Periodontol 2000. 1996 Jun;

[19] Burton Langer, Laureen Langer. Subepithelial Connective Tissue Graft Technique for Root Coverage. J Periodontol. 1985 Dec;

[20] KYU-RHIM CHUNG, MOON-YOUNG OH, SU-JIN KO. Corticotomy-Assisted Orthodontics. J Clin Orthod. 2001 May;35.

[21] B Gantes, E Rathbun, M Anholm. Effects on the periodontium following corticotomy-facilitated orthodontics. Case reports. J Periodontol. 1990 Apr;61(4).

[22] Raffaele Spena, Alfonso Caiazzo, Antonio Gracco, Giuseppe Siciliani. The use of segmental corticotomy to enhance molar distalization. J Clin Orthod. 2007 Dec;41(11).

[23] C Ochsenbein, S Ross. A reevaluation of osseous surgery. Dent Clin North Am. 1969 Jan;13(1).

[24] S SCHLUGER. Osseous resection; a basic principle in periodontal surgery. Oral Surg Oral Med Oral Pathol [Internet]. 1949 Mar; Available from: 10.1016/0030-4220(49)90363-1

[25] William Becker, Burton E Becker. Treatment of Mandibular 3-Wall Intrabony Defects by Flap Debridement and Expanded Polytetrafluoroethylene Barrier Membranes. Long-Term Evaluation of 32 Treated Patients. J Periodontol [Internet]. 1993 Nov;64. Available from: 10.1902/jop.1993.64.11s.1138

[26] Bergland Olav, Semb Gunvor, Åbyholm Frank, Borchgrevink Henrik. Secondary bone grafting and orthodontic treatment in patients with bilateral complete clefts of the lip and palate. Ann Plast Surg. 1986 Dec;460-74.

[27] Jill A. Helms, T. Michael Speidel, Kevin L. Denis. Effect of timing on long-term clinical success of alveolar cleft bone grafts. Am J Orthod Dentofac Orthop. 92(3).

[28] O Bergland, G Semb, F E Abyholm. Elimination of the residual alveolar cleft by secondary bone grafting and subsequent orthodontic treatment. Cleft Palate J. 1986 Jul;23(3):175-205.

[29] MOHAMED EL DEEB, LOUISE B. MESSER, MICHAEL W. LEHNERT, THOMAS W. HEBDA,, DANIEL E. WAITE. Canine Eruption Into Grafted Bone In Maxillary Alveolar Cleft Defects. Cleft Palate J. 1982 Jan;19(1).

[30] Hessam Nowzari, Frank Kazuo Yorita, Hsuan-Chen Chang. Periodontally accelerated osteogenic orthodontics combined with autogenous bone grafting. Compend Contin Educ Dent. 2008 May;29(4):200-6.

[31] I S Brown. The effect of orthodontic therapy on certain types of periodontal defects. I. Clinical findings. J Periodontol [Internet]. 1973 Dec;44(12). Available from: 10.1902/jop.1973.44.12.742

[32] Shigeki Ogihara, Hom-Lay Wang. Periodontal regeneration with or without limited orthodontics for the treatment of 2- or 3-wall infrabony defects. J Periodontol. 2010 Dec; 81(12).

[33] G M Kramer. Surgical alternatives in regenerative therapy of the periodontium. Int J Periodontics Restor Dent. 1992;12(1):10-31.

[34] Kokich VG, Nappen DL, Shapiro PA. Gingival contour and clinical crown length: their effect on the esthetic appearance of maxillary anterior teeth. Am J Orthod. 1984 Aug;86(2):89-94.

[35] Sterr N, Becker A. Forced eruption: biological and clinical considerations. J Oral Rehabil. 1980 Sep;7(5):395-402.

[36] Mathews DP, Kokich VG. Managing treatment for the orthodontic patient with periodontal problems. Semin Orthod. 1997 Mar;3(1):21-38. In.

[37] Rufenacht C. Structural esthetic rules. Fundam Esthet. 1992;67-132.

[38] V G Kokich. Esthetics and vertical tooth position: orthodontic possibilities. Compend Contin Educ Dent. 1997 Dec;18(12):1225-31.

Chapter 5

Genetics and Periodontal Disease: An Explicit Insight

Santo Grace Umesh, Lakshmi Ramachandran, Janani Karthikeyan and Anitha Mani

Abstract

A branch of Biology which deals with the science of hereditary influences on living organisms is termed as Genetics. There has been a broad study related to hereditary influence on human tissue linking to health and disease conditions. A vital role is played by genetics in the proper functioning, adaptive repair, regeneration and remodelling of hard and soft tissue. A major segment of genes are related to periodontal disease. Periodontal disease, being multifactorial in origin is directly or indirectly known to be caused by genetic factors also. A study on human and animals validates the concept that genetics could have influenced periodontal disorders and also plays a key role in the predisposition and progressiveness of the condition. The role played by genetics to damage the inflammatory and immune response system of the host tissues during periodontal conditions has been proved and this section will give a clear insight on the influence of genetics in this condition.

Keywords: Genetics, Periodontal disease, Hereditary influence, Polymorphism, Syndromes, Genetic study design

1. Introduction

A distinct approach is required for periodontal pathologies that produces lesions within the tooth- supporting tissues, once associated with risk factors which are complementary to systemic diseases [1]. Bacterial plaque is the prime aetiology of periodontal diseases, accelerating tissue damage. However, the role of plaque is debated when the vulnerability to periodontal diseases persist despite regular conditions. According to the majority of researchers' perspective, periodontal disease cannot occur in the absence of plaque and tartar, and also suggests that a systematic predisposition merely progresses the tissue destruction caused by microbial flora. On the other hand, few authors claim that there is no concrete evidence establishing cause-effect relationship between the nonspecific bacterial plaque and severity of tooth supporting tissue injury [2].

The host immune response system, the integrity of the tissues, humoral and cellular immunity, and certain endocrine and nutritional factors are the major factors for the development and progression of periodontal disease. Multitude of other factors are also related to periodontal diseases including age, intraoral sites that are more prone to infection and specific microbial agents such as Captosinofaga, Actinomyces naeslundi and Actinobacillus actinomycetemcomitans [2]. Apart from the host immune response system, these factors also add on to the vulnerability to periodontal disease, presenting simple to complex signs. Furthermore, the presence of associated metabolic disorders would also lead to periodontal damage [2].

Genetic elements play a vital role in influencing the inflammatory and immune response of the periodontal disease. Due to the key role played by the immune system in the pathophysiology of the disease, research is directed to identify the genetic mutation or polymorphism related to the various aspect of immunity. The result of these genetic variations might be minor or unimportant or very important and severe based on its effect and infectivity [3]. Genetic diseases are broadly classified into two entities: Simple Mendelian Disorders and Complex Genetics Disorders. Simple Mendelian Disorders are otherwise known as monogenic or single-gene disorders since they are caused by alterations of a single gene, acquired through autosomal recessive or dominant type of inheritance. Several monogenic gene disorders with biochemical defects present with severe periodontitis as one of their clinical manifestations. In these conditions, genetic alteration occurs at a single locus, producing the clinical phenotype which is responsible to cause the disease. Such a genetic alteration, that is associated with a disease phenotype in all families and there is no alternative mechanism to overcome the impact of the genetic defect, is termed as mutation [4].

Complex genetic diseases prevail in more than 1% of the population and are known to be more dominant than Simple Mendelian disorders. Being affected by environmental and lifestyle factors, complex genetic diseases occur as a result of genetic variations at multiple areas of the genes. Alterations in multiple genes, with each contributing a little to these complex genetic diseases, are called polymorphisms. Specific allele occurring in at least 1% of the population is known as genetic polymorphism. Single base mutation that replaces one nucleotide for another is said to be the simplest type of polymorphism and is termed as a single nucleotide polymorphism (SNP). Restriction fragment length polymorphism (RFLP) and simple tandem repeats (STRs), comprising of nucleotide or allele repetition are other types of polymorphism [5]. These genetic polymorphisms are not directly associated with the disease as in monogenetic disorders, however, specific alleles are found with greater incidence in the affected individuals than healthy individuals. The results prove to be true only when two different genetic variations coexist. Complex periodontal disorders are chronic, slowly progressive and are mostly of mild phenotype [5].

Variations in numerous genes encoding different proteins result in a genetic predisposition to a clinical phenotype. Environment and lifestyle play a significant role in impacting the development of complex diseases. Host response influenced by the genetic makeup is responsible for the progression of periodontal disease. Genetic defects or alterations can raise the incidence of periodontal disease. If the physiological process elicited by the gene is related to the occurrence and severity of disease, that specific gene is considered as a contributory element in periodontal disease [6]. Literature evidence reports that the genetic variants play a major role in the aetiology of syndromic and non-syndromic periodontitis.

1.1 Terminologies

1.1.1 Allele

One of two or more alternate forms of a gene or marker at a particular locus on a chromosome. (A glossary of relevant genetic terms –Dialogues in clinical neuroscience) [7].

1.1.1.1 Chromosomes

A thread-like, gene-carrying bodies in the nucleus of a cell. Chromosomes are composed primarily of DNA and protein. They are visible only under magnification during certain stages of cell division. Humans have 46 chromosomes in each somatic cell and 23 in each sex cell. (Basic principles of Genetics -Glossary of terms) [8].

1.1.1.2 Genes

Units of inheritance usually occurring at specific locations, or loci, on a chromosome. Physically, a gene is a sequence of DNA bases that specify the order of amino acids in an entire protein or, in some cases, a portion of a protein. A gene may be made up of hundreds of thousands of DNA bases. Genes are responsible for the hereditary traits in plants and animals. (Basic principles of Genetics -Glossary of terms) [8].

1.1.1.3 Genetics

The study of gene structure and action and the patterns of inheritance of traits from parent to offspring. Genetic mechanisms are the underlying foundation for evolutionary change. Genetics is the branch of science that deals with the inheritance of biological characteristics. (Basic principles of Genetics -Glossary of terms) [8].

1.1.1.4 Genotype

The genetic makeup of an individual. Genotype can refer to an organism's entire genetic makeup or the alleles at a particular locus. (Basic principles of Genetics -Glossary of terms) [8].

1.1.1.5 Monozygotic twins

Identical twins. Twins that come from the same zygote are essentially the same genetically. Differences between monozygotic twins later in life are virtually always the result of environmental influences rather than genetic inheritance. Fraternal twins may look similar but are not genetically identical. (Basic principles of Genetics -Glossary of terms) [8].

1.1.1.6 Dizygotic twins

Nonidentical twins that arise when two different eggs are fertilised by two different sperm; also called fraternal twins. (Glossary. Nature) [9].

1.1.1.7 Mutation

An alteration of genetic material such that a new variation is produced. For instance, a trait that has only one allele (A) can mutate to a new form (a). This is the only mechanism of evolution that can produce new alleles of a gene. (Basic principles of Genetics -Glossary of terms) [8].

1.1.1.8 Phenotype

The observable or detectable characteristics of an individual organism--the detectable expression of a genotype. (Basic principles of Genetics -Glossary of terms) [8].

1.1.1.9 Epigenetics

Heritable changes to DNA structure that do not alter the underlying DNA sequence, eg, DNA methylation.

1.1.1.10 Polymorphism (genetic)

The existence within a population of two or more genotypes, the rarest of which exceeds some arbitrarily low frequency (say, 1 percent); more rarely, the existence of phenotypic variation within a population, whether or not genetically based. (Glossary. Nature) [9].

1.1.1.11 Single nucleotide polymorphism (SNP)

Heritable polymorphism resulting from a single base pair change. SNPs generally have only two alleles.

1.1.1.12 Linkage

In genetics, refers to how two genes that are nearby to one another on the same chromosome are often inherited together (Glossary. Nature) [9].

1.1.1.13 Linkage disequilibrium

Describes the state of two genotypes at different loci being dependent, showing a correlation; does not require gene linkage (Glossary. Nature) [9].

1.1.1.14 Linkage equilibrium

The association of two alleles at two or more loci at the frequency predicted by their individual frequencies (Glossary. Nature) [9].

1.1.1.15 Segregational analysis

The process of fitting formal genetic models to data on expressed disease characteristics (phenotype) in biological family members in order to determine the most likely mode of inheritance for the trait or disease under study. (NCI"s Dictionary of Genetic terms) [10].

1.1.1.16 Histone modification

A histone modification is a covalent post-translational modification (PTM) to histone proteins which includes methylation, phosphorylation, acetylation, ubiquitylation, and sumoylation. The PTMs made to histones can impact gene expression by altering chromatin structure or recruiting histone modifiers. (What is epigenetics).

1.1.1.17 Linkage analysis

Study aimed at establishing linkage between genes. Today linkage analysis serves as a way of gene-hunting and genetic testing (Webster's New World medical dictionary) [11].

1.1.1.18 Concordance

The amount of similarity in phenotype between a set of individuals. May be used to refer to the presence of the same trait in both members of a pair of twins. (Molecular biology -Glossary) [12].

1.1.1.19 Discordance

Typically means that a similar trait is not shared between twin members [12].

2. Methodology

An electronic bibliographic search was carried out in three databases namely Pubmed central, Google Scholar, Ebsco, focusing on genetic studies related to periodontics. Books on genetics and periodontics were additionally referred for writing the book review.

3. Genetic study designs

The studies that show evidence of genetic predisposition to periodontitis can be grouped into four areas of research based on the statistical approaches to determine genetic components and genetic model [13].

i. Family studies.

ii. Segregation analysis.

iii. Twin studies.

iv. Population studies.

v. Linkage studies.

vi. Association studies.

3.1 Family studies

Hereditary combination of a trait or disorder will recommend genetic aetiology. Hereditary patterns may additionally indicate exposure to common environmental factors within these families. Familial aggregation could result from shared genes, shared environmental exposures and behavioural risk factors like education, socio economic grouping, oral hygiene, possible transmission of bacteria, diseases like polygenic disorder, passive smoking, exposure to pollutants and sanitation. Therefore, the complex interactions between genes and also the surroundings should even be thought-about in the analysis of familial risk for periodontic diseases [14].

3.2 Segregation analysis

They are used to study the inheritance of disease within the families. Genes are passed from parents to kids in an exceedingly foreseeable manner, and typically segregate in families as foretold by Mendel's laws [15]. Pattern of transmission of disease through generations is analysed in several families and compared with those expected under different models of inheritance to choose the best fitting model.

In this way, segregation analysis helps to identify the best model that simulates the ascertained transmission of a trait in a given population by sequential comparison with all the available models. Segregation analysis is applied by geneticists to determine whether a trait transmission belongs to Mendelian mode of genetic transmission [16].

The pattern by which disease is transmitted across generations depends on whether or not disease alleles:

- Lie on autosome/sex chromosomes.
- Dominant or Recessive.
- Fully or partially penetrant.

Genetic characteristics involving mode of transmission (e.g. autosomal, X-linked, dominant, recessive, complex, multi-locus, or random environmental), penetrance, phenocopy rates and frequencies for disease and non-disease alleles are some of the characteristics assessed in the various models. Phenotype of individual will be determined by the dominant allele. The recessive allele can be inherited only if it is located at both loci on homologous chromosomes. Penetrance refers to the possibility that a particular phenotype will rise from a genotype. Partially penetrant explains that only few individuals who inherit the disease alleles will be affected. The power of segregation analysis was dependent upon the size of population to study the observed pattern of disease.

3.2.1 Advantages

Segregation analysis helps to assess whether the disease gene is autosomal or sex linked, recessive or dominant.

3.2.2 Limitations

1. Minimal power to resolve heterogeneity (Multiple causes)
2. Cannot distinguish between genetic and environmental influences
3. Mode of inheritance among older individuals was difficult to carry out
4. Does not find or aim to find a specific gene responsible for a trait.

3.3 Twin studies

Twin studies are commonly used to study the influence of genetic and environmental factors on the complex diseases like periodontitis with multifactorial aetiology. Studying phenotypic traits of twins is a method of differentiating variations due to environmental and genetic factors [17]. Sir Francis Galton in 1875 was the first scientist to use this concept. The subject of interest in twin studies can be monozygotic or dizygotic twins.

Monozygotic twins ascend from single fertilised ovum and are therefore genetically identical and always the same sex. Dizygous twins arise from the fertilisation of two separate ovum and share one half of their descendent genes in the same way as siblings do. Concordance refers to the degree of similarity between twins in one or more characteristics whereas discordance refers to the degree of dissimilarity between twins in one or more characteristics.

Only environmental factors might account for any discordance in disease between monozygotic twins [18, 19]. Environmental and genetic variation might account for any discordance in disease between dizygotic twins. Presuming that the environmental influence is constant, the effects of excess shared genes in monozygotic twins measures the difference in discordance between monozygotic (MZ) and dizygotic (DZ) twins [20, 21].

For binary traits (present or absent), a genetic effect is inferred if the positive concordance rate, or percentage of twin pairs in which both twins are affected, is greater for MZ than DZ twins.

There are two types of twin studies:

i. Classic twin study- Monozygotic and dizygotic twins are reared together and compared.

ii. Study in which monozygotic twins are reared apart- This study shows the effects of shared genes without the confounding effects of a common family environment. Any similarities between both of them will be attributed to their shared genes and dissimilarities will be because of environmental factors.

Heritability, which refers to the proportion of phenotypic variation attributed to genetic variation, can be evaluated efficiently by twin data. 50% heritability clearly states that half of phenotypic variance in the population is attributed to genetic variance and it does not imply that a child of an affected parent has a 50% chance of inheriting the disease.

It was proposed that 38–82% of the population variance for probing depth (PD), attachment loss (AL) and dental plaque may be attributed to genetic factors in a study involving 110 pairs of adult twins [22]. A successive study on 64 monozygotic and 53 dizygotic pairs of adult twins disclosed the fact that genetic variance contributes to almost half of the variance in disease pattern in the population. From the results of the study, it was concluded that MZ twins were more alike than DZ twins for all clinical parameters [23].

Therefore, the difference in concordance between MZ and DZ twins for a specific phenotype could be used to evaluate the relative contribution of genes (heredity) and environmental factors to a disease and analysing disease presentation in twins is an essential first step in this process. Though twin studies overcame the drawbacks of segregation analysis, few such studies have been conducted because of the inadequacy of such twins.

3.4 Population studies

Environmental or behavioural risk factors for a disease are usually first detected in significant epidemiological or population-based studies. A genetic polymorphism is the long-time manifestation in a population of two or more genotypes that could not be maintained by frequent mutation.

The frequencies of polymorphisms of candidate genes can be compared between diseased individuals and controls [4]. It can be proved that the candidate gene determines the vulnerability to disease when there is a clear cut difference in the frequency of a specific polymorphism, between a case group and a control group. In this way, pathogenesis, causal heterogeneity of disease process and individuals most at risk for the disease can be interpreted well [24, 25].

In chronic periodontitis, no evidence of any simple pattern of genetic transmission that would support an etiologic role for a single gene mutation is demonstrated. In contrast to simple genetic diseases that may be caused by a single genetic mutation, the additive effect of multiple genes is a determinant of disease susceptibility in complex diseases such as chronic periodontitis [14].

3.5 Linkage studies

Linkage analysis is a technique used to map the gene responsible for a trait to a specific position on a chromosome. These studies are based on the information that genes that are located closely on the same chromosome incline to have inherited together as a unit. Such genes are said to be linked and defy Mendel's law of independent assortment.

The distance between two allele at different loci will determine whether they will recombine. This is termed as recombination or crossover event. There is 50% chance that any two maternal or paternal alleles will recombine and be transmitted together to an offspring. However, alleles at nearby loci are linked and they tend to segregate together.

Linkage study necessitates use of very expensive DNA markers which was acceptable only after learning strong evidence of a genetic basis for a trait using segregation analysis or family aggregation analysis. By identifying the genetic markers that are associated with the disease causing alleles, the researchers can modify the location of a disease allele. Inheritance of a disease can be established if the distance between marker and disease allele is within 20–30 centimo grams (cM). In humans, 1 cM represents approximately 1 million nucleotide bases.

In this way, segregation of a trait in a manner consistent with linkage to a known genetic marker can be tested. Once the linkage is detected, the gene responsible for the trait can be placed in the vicinity of the linked genetic polymorphism since the exact chromosomal location of the genetic marker is known. Hence the genetic basis of disease is proved by linkage. Linkage is usually used as an initial step to identify the approximate location of a gene of interest, allowing the successive studies to determine the mutation responsible for a disease trait.

Linkage studies usually start by identifying markers (Single Nucleotide Polymorphisms) on a section of chromosome and then narrowing down the region until the gene of interest is found. DNA markers that are located proximal to a disease gene will be inclined to be inherited together with the disease gene. The closer a marker is to the disease gene, the closer the linkage and the more likely it is that they will be inherited together.

Linkage studies use sets of families, containing multiple affected individuals. Genotypes are determined for affected and unaffected family members, and complex statistical models are used to decide whether marker allele and disease co-segregate in the families under a given inheritance model.

Linkage is calculated using a LOD (Logarithm of odds) score. It is described as the ratio of probability that the disease and the marker loci are linked rather than unlinked. Supporting linkage gives a LOD score of +3 (1000:1) whereas, absence of linkage denotes a score of −2. Boughman et al. was first to assess the linkage between dentinogenesis imperfecta and aggressive periodontitis [26].

Marker linked to disease allele within a family may not be linked with disease in the population, which implies that same marker allele need not be transmitted with the disease allele in all affected families. However, Allelic associations (which is discussed below) occur when the same marker allele is linked to disease in multiple families.

3.5.1 Drawbacks

- Linkage studies have been successful only in identifying the genetic basis of simple Mendelian traits, where mutation of a single gene can cause a disease.

DOI: http://dx.doi.org/10.5772/intechopen.99266

Nevertheless, Linkage studies of complex diseases are not successful since complex diseases are due to the combined effect of multiple genes of minor effect and each gene contribute a small amount to the disease phenotype [27, 28].

- It has extremely low statistical power for diseases in which there is extensive heterogeneity among different families that have different combinations of vulnerable genes and environmental exposures.

3.6 Association studies

Associations indicate that the presence of an allele confers risk for disease within a specific environment. Allele association helps to identify whether the frequency of an allele is considerably increased or decreased in a particular disease. The difference between association studies and genetic linkage is that association studies compare a population of affected individuals with control population whereas, the latter is demonstrable only in families or siblings.

Therefore, Association studies involve candidate gene approach, a gene mapping approach that tests whether one allele of a gene appears more frequently in patients with disease than in subjects without the disease. Candidate genes are selected based on their reasonable role in disease process such as producing a protein that is important in disease pathogenesis.

Linkage disequilibrium is a term used when the same marker allele is linked with disease in multiple families. Frequency of allele at a given locus is compared between patients with disease and healthy subjects to test this association. Biologic link between the disease and an allele cannot be confirmed through association. Association might result due to few environmental factors causing both the marker and the disease to rise in the population, or due to a difference in the racial or ethnic makeup of the cases and controls, or from chance alone [29]. True linkage disequilibrium refers to a situation when marker and disease allele are placed close to each other on chromosomes and the chances of disease are more.

On the whole, this population-based approach compares marker allele frequencies between affected and unaffected individuals, using a standard case–control design. When a positive association is found, few interpretations are made: [30].

- Associated allele is considered as the disease-predisposing allele.
- Associated allele is in linkage disequilibrium with the exact disease-predisposing locus.
- Association arise out of population stratification.
- Association is a sampling, or statistical, artefact.

Numerous case control studies are reported in which genotype frequencies of an inherited DNA variant for a group of periodontitis cases are statistically compared to periodontally healthy control subjects. If the genotype frequencies vary so much that the results are very unlikely to occur by coincidence, it is assumed that the genotype is more common in cases than controls and is associated with high disease risk.

3.6.1 Advantages

Association studies are beneficial for discovery of inherited genetic variation important for a wide range of complex diseases including diabetes, cardiovascular diseases, metabolic disorders, obesity and mental illness.

3.6.2 Disadvantages

- Alleles that can be used to predict disease in one population may not be useful in other populations or even in the same population when exposed to extremely different environments. In the presence of pathogens, individuals with the low response allele develop disease. On the other hand, no relationship may exist between the disease and this allele in populations where the particular bacteria is absent.
- Low power to evaluate small genetic effects
- Small presentation of actual causal or rare variants
- Non-consideration of prior mechanistic or biological information [31]

3.7 Evidence for the role of genetic variants in periodontitis

The above mentioned studies demonstrate that different genetic loci are capable of causing the disease in dominant and recessive ways [32]. Few of the genes responsible are autosomal whereas others are X-linked. These factors account for the different observed modes of transmission (**Tables 1–4**).

Author	Study	Results
Melnick et al., 1976 [32]	Mode of inheritance for Aggressive Periodontitis among Caucasians and African-Americans	X linked inheritance-preponderance of female probands
Saxen, 1984 [33]	Mode of inheritance for Aggressive Periodontitis among Finnish population	Autosomal recessive mode of inheritance
Marazita et al., 1994 [34]	Largest US study among African-Americans to evaluate the mode of inheritance for aggressive periodontitis	Autosomal Dominant mode with penetrance of about 80%
Schenkein, 1994 [35]	Subjects with one AP disease allele and two copies of the high IgG2 response allele develops Localised Aggressive periodontitis Subjects with one AP disease allele and one copy of high IgG2 response allele develops widespread disease since their IgG2 response to LPS would be less robust.	Aggressive Periodontitis disease and IgG2 responsiveness to bacterial LPS segregate independently as dominant and codominant trails

Table 1.
Segregation analysis.

Author	Study	Results
Corey et al., 1992 [36]	Questionnaire survey for several thousand adult twin pairs about the history of periodontal disease	Concordance rate was greater in MZ twins than DZ twins.
Michalowicz 1991 [22]	Independent twin studies at Minnesota and Virginia in which the relative contribution of environmental and host genetic factors to clinical measures of periodontal disease were examined	Significant heritable component for gingivitis, PD, CAL, plaque. 38–82% of the population variance for these periodontal measures of disease may be attributed to genetic factors.

Table 2.
Twin studies.

Author	Study	Results
Boughman et al.,1986 [26]	First to report linkage of Localised Aggressive Periodontitis and a specific chromosomal region.	Aggressive periodontitis segregates with Dentinogenesis imperfecta. Localised to long arm of chromosome 4 near the gene for dentinogenesis imperfecta
Li Y et al., 2004 [37]	Study conducted on 4 families with Localised Aggressive Periodontitis	Aggressive Periodontitis has been linked to a marker on choromosome 1(1q25) with LOD-3.48.
Tabeta K et al., 2009 [38]	Linkage disequilibrium block analysis- SNPs and Microsatellites in chromosome 19	A single microsatellite marker allele 17 of 1902 G31 on chromosome 19- associated with severe chronic periodontitis

Table 3.
Linkage studies.

Author	Study	Results
Korman et al., 1997 [39]	Composite IL-1 genotype consisting atleast one copy of the rare allele at both an IL- 1 α and IL -1β loci was associated with severe periodontitis in North European adults.	Association-18.9 Genotype positive nonsmokers were 6.8 times likely to have severe periodontal disease.
Gore et al., 1998 [40]	Study conducted to analyse composite genotype in Caucasians	More rare IL-1β sites were in linkage disequilibrium,ie. IL-1 β allele was found to be more prevalent in chronic periodontitis than the composite genotype.
Kobayashi et al., 1997 [41]	Tested association between neutrophil IgG receptor FcγR polymorphisms and Chronic periodontitis in a Japanese population	Association was found with FcγRIII-NA2 allele and it was more prevalent in those with recurrent disease.
Engebretson et al., 1999 [42]	Study conducted on periodontitis patients who were positive for composite IL-1 genotype in US population	Elevated levels of IL-1β in GCF
Galbraith et al., 1998 [43]	TNF genotypes were determined in 32 Caucasian patients with chronic periodontitis and 32 orally healthy matched controls, and correlated with TNF- alpha production by oral polymorphonuclear leukocytes	No association between Chronic Periodontitis and TNF- α polymerisation
Sofaer et al., 1990 [44]	Study conducted on patients with Aggressive periodontitis (AP)	HLA A-9 and B15 antigens were constantly associated with AP. The risk of disease was 1.5 to 3.5 times greater than those lacking these antigen
Terazaki et al., 1975 [45]	Study conducted on patients with Aggressive periodontitis (AP)	HLA- A2 antigen appears to be less prevalent in patients with AP than controls suggesting a protective role
Katz et al., 1987 [46]	Study conducted on patients with Chronic and Aggressive periodontitis (AP)	MHC class II DR4 antigen were at increased risk of type of DM 1 related complications including periodontitis DR4 antigen was more prevalent in patients with AP disease than controls

Table 4.
Association studies.

4. Genetic polymorphisms and periodontal disease

A polymorphism is a form of genetic variant that appears in at least 1% of a population and evolves from mutation. 90% of polymorphisms come from Single Nucleotide Polymorphisms (SNPs) where a single base of one nucleotide is replaced with another. In majority of SNP that occur in genes, the protein produced remains unaffected, but have an effect on the gene product. Since all forms of periodontal disorders are linked with bacterial infections, outlining the relative roles of genes and environmental factors in these complex disorders is a challenge [47]. In case of chronic periodontitis, studies on twin adults imply that a sizable proportion of the population variance for periodontal measures such as pocket depth, attachment loss, and bone loss might be endorsed to genetics. Early onset periodontitis is often genetic, and the likelihood of inheriting periodontitis is high, as indicated by genetic studies [48].

A large part of in vitro and in vivo analyses [49] of human tissues as well as studies in animals strongly confirms that cytokines play a key role at all stages of the immune response in periodontal disorder. The various genetic polymorphisms associated with periodontal diseases are shown in (**Figure 1**).

4.1 Inflammatory and anti-inflammatory cytokines

4.1.1 Interleukin-1

IL-1 gene polymorphisms were the first described genetic markers related to periodontal disease in 1997 [10]. The three cytokines originally defined as the members of the IL-1 family were IL-1α and IL-1β, are the major agonistic molecules, whereas IL-1Ra, a biological antagonist. These functionally similar molecules are encoded on separate genes in the same region of chromosome 2. SNP's were found in IL-1 gene cluster, a C to T transition at nucleotide: 889 in the IL-1α and the second at +3954 of IL-1β gene. Occurrence of allele 2 of the IL-1B +3953 SNP was significantly increased in patients with advanced periodontal disorder [50–54].

Dental Implants: Investigations in individuals with polymorphisms of IL-1α and IL-1β genes with IL-1β – 511 2/2 genotype showed evidence of a substantially higher incidents of marginal bone loss [55].

Intrabony defects: Impact of IL-1 gene polymorphism on clinical and radiographic healing results in patients treated with Guided Tissue Regeneration (GTR) therapy [56] did not reveal any statistical variations between IL-1 + and IL-1 – patients.

4.1.2 Interleukin-2

It is established that – 330 (T → G) polymorphism in IL-2 gene is related to acute and vital role in pathogenesis of periodontitis [57].

4.1.3 Interleukin-4

Study of IL-4 gene polymorphisms in the intron 2 and in the promoter positions (PP+ and IP+) showed no link with periodontal disease exposure.

4.1.4 Interleukin 6

IL-6 in intron 2 and in the promoter positions (PP- and IP) gene polymorphisms in chronic periodontitis suggested that −572 G/C polymorphisms of IL-6 gene may be one of the protecting factors connected with lower susceptibility to chronic periodontal disease [50–53].

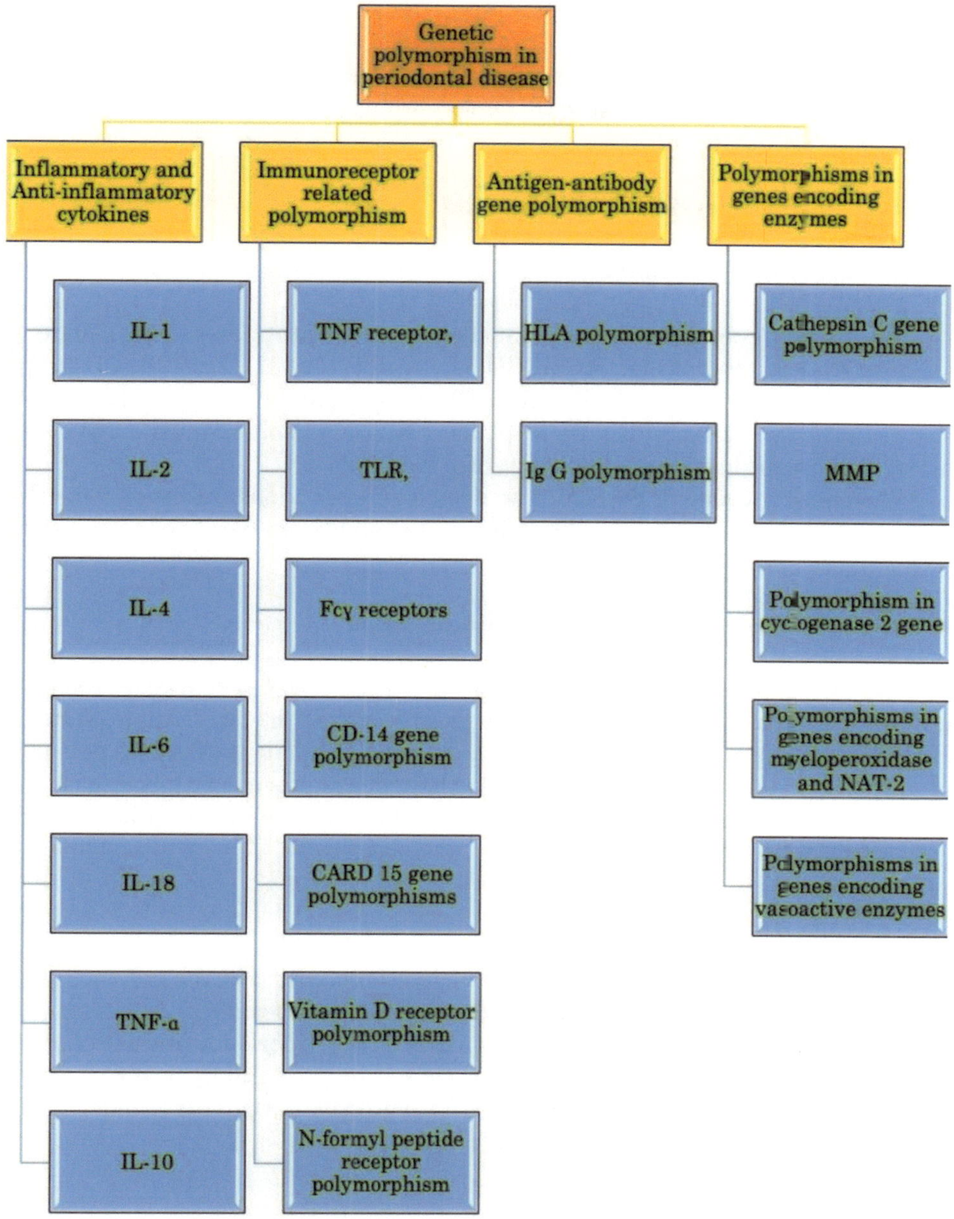

Figure 1.
Flowchart showing the various genetic polymorphisms associated with periodontal disease.

4.1.5 Tumour necrosis factor-α

Study to explore 4 polymorphisms in TNF- α gene which are all transitions from G to A, 3 in the promoter positions: – 376, – 308, – 238 and at position +489, failed to be identified as susceptibility or severity factors in periodontitis.

4.1.6 Interleukin-10

Three SNPs in the promoter regions of IL10 genes, a G to A transition, at position – 1087, C to T transition at 819, and a C to A transition at 592 have been linked with altered synthesis of IL10.

4.1.7 Interleukin 18

Six different IL-18 gene polymorphism (–656, –607, –137, +113, +127, and codon 35/3) were investigated and none of the polymorphisms were linked to destructive periodontal disease [38, 44].

4.2 Immunoreceptor related polymorphism

4.2.1 Fcγ receptor polymorphisms

The phagocytes harbour the Fc-gamma receptor which attaches to IgG. There are three broad classes of FcR: FcãRI (CD 64), FcãR II (CD 32), FcãR III (CD 16) in chromosome 1. Of which FcãR IIIa and FcãR IIIb, is found to be frequently associated with chronic periodontitis. FcãR IIIb has a NA1-NA2 polymorphism. NA1 is a more efficient opsono-phagocytic agent than NA2 [58].

When one or several of FcγR-mediated leukocyte functions are less or over efficient due to polymorphisms, it is likely that vulnerability or severity of periodontal disease is seen [46, 47].

4.2.2 Toll-like receptors (TLR-2,-4) gene polymorphism

These are signal molecules essential for the cellular response to bacterial cell wall components. TLR 2 exhibits polymorphism (Arg to Thr at 677, Arg to Gly at 753) which alters their ability to respond to cell wall components. Polymorphism of TLR4 (Asp 299 Arg 677 Trp; Arg753 Gln) have been known to be linked with impaired Lipopolysaccharide (LPS) signal transduction. Their relationship has still not been established [48].

4.2.3 CD14 gene polymorphism

The transcriptional activity of the CD 14 gene is enhanced by the presence of R-allele in the promoter region at position –260(–159). Research in Caucasian population revealed CD14–260 polymorphism in chronic periodontitis with no major link. A higher frequency of the N –allele and the N/N genotype of CD14–1359 polymorphism were observed in patients with aggressive periodontitis and in subjects with severe periodontal disorder [37, 41].

4.2.4 CARD 15 gene polymorphisms

The 3020insC and 2104 C > T polymorphisms seen in CARD15 (NOD2) gene results in decreased stimulation of nuclear factor-kappa B, thereby leads to alteration in the gene expression of pro inflammatory cytokine genes and diminished production of cytokines. However there has been no further established role for CARD 15 from studies in Caucasians [52].

4.2.5 Polymorphism of RANK gene

RANKL and its receptor RANK are the key elements reported to cause increased bone resorption in periodontal disease through osteoclast differentiation and activation of nuclear factor-B (RANK), RANK ligand (RANKL), and osteoprotegrin (OPG). Association studies show no significant link of the SNPs with AgP in Japanese population.

4.2.6 N-formyl peptide receptor polymorphism

FMLP receptor has a high affinity variant (FPR1) which binds with FMLP receptors of microbial cells triggering chemotaxis, degranulation and superoxide production which are found to be disrupted in genetically modified periodontitis. Polymorphisms were noted at the nt329T-C (codon 110 phenylalanine-serine), and at the nt378C-G (codon 126 cysteine-tryptophan) in the 583 bp interval of FMLP receptor gene. Coincidentally this is found to be significantly linked to the Agp phenotype in Afro-American patients [17, 18].

4.2.7 Vitamin D receptor (VDR) polymorphisms

Vitamin D receptor gene polymorphism has influence on bone mineral density and turnover. Studies proved vitamin D receptor (VDR) gene is localised in chromosome 12 with a group of polymorphisms: BsmI, ApaI and TaqI and relationship between TaqI VDR gene polymorphisms and periodontitis.

4.3 Antigen–antibody gene polymorphism

4.3.1 HLA genetics

The MHC genes are the most polymorphic genes present in the genome of every living organism. Research implied that patients with HLA-DRB1*1501-DQB1*0602 genotype may have accelerated T cell response and are thereby prone to periodontitis.

4.3.2 Immunoglobulin g2 variations

IgG molecules constitute genetically strong variants in the gamma heavy chains, termed Gm allotypes. Patients with rapidly progressing periodontitis with positive Gm shows higher antibodies [54].

4.4 Polymorphism in genes encoding enzymes

4.4.1 Cathepsin C gene polymorphism

Cathepsin C is a lysosomal protease in neutrophils and macrophages identified in chromosome 11, responsible for periodontal disease in young children termed as prepubertal periodontitis [51, 52].

4.4.2 Matrix metalloproteinases(MMP) polymorphisms

MMP-1 is an important mediator of connective tissue destruction in periodontal disease. A single nucleotide polymorphism in the promoter position of - 1607 bp of MMP-1 gene a, 5′-GGA-3′, instead of 5′-GAT-3′ has been identified to be linked with higher threat of generalised aggressive periodontitis [58].

4.4.3 Polymorphisms in cyclogenase –2 gene

PGE2 is a significant mediator of tissue destruction, catalysed by COX-2. A SNP of COX-2 in the chromosome 9q32–33. This modifies the expression of the COX-2 gene and polymorphism of -765G to C is linked with lesser risk for periodontitis.

4.4.4 Polymorphisms in genes encoding myeloperoxidase (MPO) and N-acetyl transferase (NAT-2)

A SNP in the promoter position of −1607 bp of MMP-1 gene a, 5′-GGA-3′, instead of 5′-GAT-3′ has been learned to be connected with increased risk of generalised aggressive periodontitis. A link between bone density loss in periodontal disease and polymorphism of NAT2 have been reported [59].

4.4.5 Polymorphisms in genes encoding vasoactive enzymes

The study of genotypes between affected and healthy showed the presence of lymphotoxin-á (TNF-â), angiotensin- converting enzyme and endothelin-1(ET-1) polymorphism with link to three-locus combination [41, 60].

5. Periodontal diseases as a manifestation of systemic genetic disorders

Certain systemic disorders predispose the patient's susceptibility to acquire periodontal disease, which may present clinically in a chronic or an aggressive form. The *involved pathogenesis includes* modifications in the immune, endocrine and connective tissue status of the individual. These changes eventually result in the occurrence of syndromes with periodontal disease either as a primary manifestation or by aggravating a pre-existing condition associated with the presence of local factors. The alterations in the immune system may be noted at cellular and/or humoral level. Lymphocytes play a pivotal role in driving the immune response, and a defect or absence of one or more lineages may result in fatal conditions like leukaemia or Acquired immune-deficiency syndrome [61]. Neutrophil defects in turn may be of a qualitative (altered chemotaxis and phagocytosis) or quantitative nature (neutropenia, agranulocytosis), and both predispose to rapid and severe periodontal destruction.

A high susceptibilty to develop periodontitis has been associated with conditions such as Down syndrome (trisomy 21), Chediak-Higashi syndrome and Papillon-Lefèvre syndrome. These subjects present with an increased incidence of infections with a plausibility owing to a diminished expression of surface glycoproteins required for bacterial adhesion [62]. Other connective tissue disorders, also induce an elevation to periodontal inflammation mostly linked with plaque and in some cases an overstated response relatively disproportionate to the amount of microbial plaque present.

5.1 Unleashing the underlying mechanism

Inorder to understand the pathogenesis of Genetic diseases, they have been broadly classified as,

a. Connective tissue deformities: eg Marfan syndrome, Ehler-Danlos syndrome.

b. Immune related alterations: eg severe congenital neutropenia (SCN) or infantile genetic agranulocytosis or Kostmann syndrome (IGA), Chediak-Higiashi syndrome, Down syndrome, Papillon-Lefèvre syndrome, hyperimmunoglobulinemia E syndrome [61].

5.2 Systemic and periodontal manifestations of common genetic disorders

5.2.1 Connective tissue deformities

5.2.1.1 Marfan syndrome

Mutation of a gene encoding for fibril-1 present in chromosome 15 marks a defect in the synthesis of a glycoprotein forming part of the connective tissue matrix. This causes defects in a series of locations such as the ocular lens suspensory ligament, blood vessel walls and, apparently, the periodontal ligament [62].

Periodontal manifestations:

The mode of periodontal pathogenesis in these syndromes can be understood by connective tissue modifications which generates increased vulnerability to periodontal inflammation and bone resorption. Despite the co-existence of a similar background alteration, the manifestations of periodontal disease vary in their presentation in each of the syndromes. For instance, Marfan syndrome exhibit both chronic and severe form of disease with patterns of horizontal and vertical bone resorption, in accordance to the presence of bacterial plaque. However, tooth mobility has been shown to be a sequel to periodontitis, and is not endorsed to the primary condition of the syndrome [62, 63].

5.2.1.2 Ehler-Danlos syndrome

Ehlers-Danlos syndrome (EDS) comprises a group of genetic diseases involving the connective tissue characterised by mutations in the genes responsible for the collagen biosynthesis. The clinical expressions of EDS include increased tissue fragility, hypermobility of joints, and hyperextensibility of skin [64].

Periodontal manifestations

In EDS, periodontal disease can be linked with syndromes type I, VII, III, or IV. Type I EDS has *increased predisposition to periodontal disease, whereas type VIII manifests as early onset periodontitis, with premature loss of permanent teeth, fragility of the mucosa leading to bleeding gums and oral mucosa The postulated mechanism is a defect in type III collagen, amounting to a total of periodontal junction. Moreover, a relationship has been found to Fusobacterium nucleatum, which could be isolated from the active affected sites* [65].

5.2.2 Immune related conditions

The immune conditions contemplated in the above classification are all primary immune deficiencies caused by a decrease in neutrophil presence, or by modifications in the functions of these cells – as in the above cited syndromes. These conditions predispose patients to bacterial and fungal infections in childhood, because the decrease in neutrophil presence alters the host defence capacity. Additionally, a drop is seen in the production of granulocyte colony stimulating factors [66, 67]. Let us discuss some significant disorders.

5.2.2.1 Chediak-Higiashi syndrome

Chediak-Higiashi syndrome is supplemented by leukocyte modification, basically limited to the lysosomes, which destroy melanosomes producing oculocutaneous albinism. Affected patients also present mental retardation, and neutropenia additionally may also be observed – with altered LA.

5.2.2.2 Down syndrome

Down syndrome or trisomy 21 results because of chromosomal abnormality that causes peculiar physical changes, with co-existing mental retardation and other systemic alterations. The immune changes described in Down syndrome are linked to function of WBCs, responsible for the defensive mechanisms in periodontal tissues [68, 69].

5.2.2.3 Papillon-Lefèvre syndrome

Papillon-Lefèvre syndrome is classically manifested as palmoplantar erythematous hyperkeratosis along with periodontal disease. The proposed mechanism is linked to a mutation of the gene encoding for cathepsin C, which generates a lysosomal protein implicated to modify the host immune response, inflammatory response and extracellular matrix function with significant changes in the palmar, plantar and gingival epithelium [64]. Hyperimmunoglobulinemia E (HE) consists of an increase in serum immunoglobulin E (IgE). This in turn leads to a series of systematic variations with involvement of the skin, facial malformations and increased vulnerability to staphylococcal infections [70, 71].

5.3 Periodontal manifestations of immune related disorders

In neutrophil disorders, the notable reduction in the amount of neutrophils tends to disregulate the host defence capacity, causing periodontal disease to manifest at a younger age. Gingival inflammation, aggressive periodontal tissue destruction, edema, pocket formation and tooth mobility are common presentations. This clinical representation is much similar to prepuberal or rapidly progressive periodontitis with premature loss of the deciduous teeth [66, 68, 72].

5.3.1 Chediak-Higiashi syndrome

Chediak-Higiashi syndrome manifests as early occurrence of periodontitis with premature exfoliation of both dentitions. The bone resorption patterns may be local or generalised, and are linked to associated inflammation. The disorder is associated with anaerobic flora, due to the amble presence of purulent processes. The abundant presence of spirochetes in the locations with inflammation and high proteolytic activity, which facilitates bacterial adherence further explains the pathosis. Adding to this, the co-existence of lysosomal modifications and defective chemotaxis in neutrophils gives rise to very rapidly progressing periodontitis that inclines to be recurrent and is refractory to antibiotic treatment [68].

5.3.2 Down syndrome

Down syndrome is characterised by aggressive and generalised periodontitis, with subsequent damage of the supporting tissues and loss of teeth at an early age. Eight percent of Down syndrome children suffer periodontal lesions by 12 years of age [73]. The rate of occurence of periodontal disease in this population ranges from 60–100% in young adults under 30 years of age [70]. The co existence of immune deficiency, inadequate control of bacterial plaque, deficient masticatory function, early ageing and alterations in dental anatomy (short roots) predispose or aggravate the progression of periodontal disease [74, 75].

In patients with higher level of mental retardation, difficulties are observed with relation to oral hygiene maintenance. Oral health care needs to be emphasised

Syndrome	Mode of inheritance	Defect	Function of normal gene	Oral & periodontal manifestation
Severe congenital neutropenia type 1	Autosomal dominant	Neutrophil elastase gene (ela2)- 19p13.36	The products of elastase gene degrade membrane protein a of bacterial cell wall.	Early age periodontitis similar to pre pubertal periodontitis
Severe congenital neutropenia type ii	Autosomal dominant	Growth factor independent gene (GFi 1) 1p226 GFi 1 gene	Function to replace ela2	Early age periodontitis6
Severe congenital neutropenia type iii	Autosomal recessive	Ar hcls1 associated protein x1 (hax1)- 1q21.36	Controls development of neutrophils	Early age periodontitis6
Hiam-munk syndrome	Autosomal recessive	Cathepsin c- ctsc 602365- on chromosome 11q14.6.7,14	Degrading proteins and activation proenzymes in immune cells.	aggressive periodontitis
Phosphatasia	Autosomal dominant or recessive	Alkaline phosphatase liver/bone/ kidney (alpl)-1p36.1-p3412,13,15	Maintains normal level of alkaline phosphatase aggressive periodontitis	Premature loss of primary teeth Aggressive periodontitis
Kindler syndrome	Autosomal recessive	Kindlin 1(kind 1)- 20p136,19	Normal basement membrane, cell to contact	Aggressive periodontitis in primary and permanent dentition.
Infantile genetic agranulocytosis	Autosomal recessive	Elane (formerly ela2) gene on chromosome 19p13.36,7,8 deficiency of Il-37,	Synthesis of neutrophil elastase, a peptide antibiotic present in neutrophils	Aggressive periodontitis
Hyper ige job's syndrome (hie)	Autosomal. recessive	7q216,12,16	Regulation of IgE	Opportunistic infections, periodontitis and oral ulcerations
Familial and cyclic neutropenia	Autosomal dominant	Elane mutation	Regulating the number of circulating neutrophils	Oral ulcers, Gingival inflammation, Severe periodontitis
Down syndrome	Autosomal dominant	Trisomy chromosome 21	Normal chemotaxis and phagocytosis	Gingivitis, Necrotizing ulcerative gingivitis, Severe periodontitis, Tooth mobility

Syndrome	Mode of inheritance	Defect	Function of normal gene	Oral & periodontal manifestation
Leukocyte adhesion deficiency syndrome	Autosomal. recessive	Integrin b2 (itgb2)- 21q22.37,9,11	Adhesion receptors of the white blood cells and phagocytosis	*Type 1:* severe gingival inflammation, Rapidly progressive periodontitis, *Type 2:* chronic severe periodontitis
Papillon-lefèvre syndrome	Autosomal recessive	Cathepsin c gene11q14-q216,14,17 mutation of gene encoding for cathepsin-c,	Neutrophil function	Aggressive periodontitis, Premature loss of teeth
Chédiak-higashi syndrome	Autosomal recessive	Mutation in lyst gene Lysosomal trafficking regulator gene (lyst)-1q42.1-q42.26,7,14	Transport of vesicles to and from the neutrophil lysosyme9,11	Oral ulcerations, Severe gingivitis Early-onset periodontitis
Histiocytosis syndromes	Unknown	Abnormal proliferation of bone marrow-derived histiocytes	—	Periodontitis, Alveolar bone loss replaced by soft tissue, Oral ulceration, Premature loss of teeth
Glycogen storage disease	Autosomal recessive	*Type 1b:* deficiency of glucose-6-phosphate translocase	Regulation of glycogen breakdown	Oral ulcers, Hyperplastic gingiva, Periodontal infections, Prolonged bleeding
Severe congenital neutropenia	Autosomal dominant	Elane and hax1 mutations	Maintainance of circulating neutrophil	Gingival inflammation, Increased probing depth, Severe alveolar bone loss in both dentitions
Cohen syndrome	Autosomal recessive	Mutation in the vps13b gene	Functional vps13b protein.	Early adult periodontitis
Ehlers-danlos syndrome (type iv and viii)	Autosomal dominant	*Type iv:* mutation in *type iii* collagen *Type viii:* mutation in chromosome 12p13	Synthesis of type iii collagen	Severe periodontitis Prolonged bleeding Delayed healing

Table 5.
Comprehensive tabulation of genetic disorders and their periodontal manifestations [44, 61, 62].

in order to avoid the accumulation of plaque leading to initiation of the disease [76–78]. The presence of defective neutrophil chemotaxis, leads to progressive periodontitis as observed in juvenile periodontitis. Concurrently, it has been reported that the B cells,T cells, and monocytes, also illustrate functional defects. The periodontal destruction is directly proportional to the degree of alteration in functional chemotaxis. The mechanism mounting for the dysfunction is attributed to a decrease in the number of cell surface receptors, and diminished levels of zinc and some vitamins in serum [70].

5.3.3 Papillon-Lefèvre syndrome

Papillon-Lefèvre syndrome presents as aggressive periodontal inflammation with the premature loss of both primary and permanent dentitions. The underlying mechanism involved are due to immune modifications apart from alterations in the gingival tissues along with the notable presence of *Actinobacillus actinomycetemcomitans* [72].

5.3.4 Hyperimmunoglobulinemia E syndrome

Hyperimmunoglobulinemia E syndrome manifests with overhiked susceptibility to infections and thus contributing to the development of periodontitis. The process involved here is thought to be associated with a deficient host cellular and humoral immune response, comprising of an inadequate neutrophil chemotaxis secondary to alteration in the regulation of T cell cytokines. The rapid spike in circulating IgE leads to a reduced production of gamma-interferon, which intervenenes with anti-inflammatory and bone resorption-inhibiting processes. Thereby, the heightened inflammatory and resorptive phenomena noted in these patients, gives rise to early and advanced periodontitis. This disorder is associated with abundance of pathogenic microflora (*P. gingivalis, T. denticola, E. corrodens*) that results in severe periodontal damage in adults and in children [73]. The syndromes, mode of inheritance, function of responsible gene and periodontal manifestations are given in **Table 5**.

6. Future perspectives

At least 50% of periodontitis vulnerability is attributed to heredity or genetic factors [20]. Clinical observations and scientific studies have demonstrated that the heredity of a host response pattern may be an important susceptibility factor in developing periodontal diseases [20, 79, 80]. Added information from new technologies, such as micro-arrays and DNA-sequencing, lead to the identification of specific genetic, environmental, and behavioural factors that influence periodontitis susceptibility [81].

In order to enhance the therapeutic management of periodontal disease, we must not only be able to identify genetic determinants, but also learn to modify, control or modulate the host response either by stimulating a desired immune response, or by decreasing the activating factors of bone resorption,both of which hinders the progression of the disease by [82–84].

7. Concluding remarks

At present, the clinical application of the effect of genetics in periodontics is minimal. Despite several researches revealing association of candidate gene polymorphisms with periodontal disease, lacunae lies owing to co-existence of multiple etiotrophic factors and the plausible role of epigenetics in the periodontal disease severity. Future research shall be directed towards multiple genes, their interactions and role of epigenetics in modifying the periodontal etiopathogenesis.

Conflict of interest

The authors declare no conflict of interest.

Author details

Santo Grace Umesh*, Lakshmi Ramachandran, Janani Karthikeyan
and Anitha Mani
SRM Dental College, Ramapuram, SRM Institute of Science and Technology,
Chennai, Tamil Nadu, India

*Address all correspondence to: grace.santo@gmail.com

References

[1] Fernández PB, Portillo GM. Tratamiento odontológico en pacientes especiales. Laboratorios Normon; 2004.

[2] Wilton JM, Griffiths GS, Curtis MA, Maiden MF, Gillett IR, Wilson DT, Sterne JA, Johnson NW. Detection of high-risk groups and individuals for periodontal diseases: Systemic predisposition and markers of general health. Journal of clinical Periodontology. 1988 Jul;15(6):339-46.

[3] Tarannum F, Faizuddin M. Effect of gene polymorphisms on periodontal diseases. Indian journal of human genetics. 2012 Jan;18(1):9.

[4] Taba Jr M, Souza SL, Mariguela VC. Periodontal disease: a genetic perspective. Brazilian oral research. 2012;26(spe1):32-8.

[5] Masamatti DS, Kumar A, Dodwad V. Role of Genetics in Periodontal Diseases. Journal of Innovative Dentistry. 2011;1(2).

[6] Bali D, Pandit N, Kathuria R, Bali A. Genetics and aggressive periodontal disease: an update review. J Oral Heal Community Dent. 2012 May;6:97-101.

[7] Morris-Rosendahl DJ. A glossary of relevant genetic terms. Dialogues in clinical neuroscience. 2010 Mar;12(1):116.

[8] Martínez Mir A, Christiano AM. Basic principles of genetics.

[9] Gellner JL, Weaver WL. A Glossary of Genetic Terms. Dick. J. Envtl. L. & Pol'y. 1993;3:119

[10] NCI"s Dictionary of Genetic terms https://www.cancer.gov/publications/dictionaries/genetics-dictionary/def/segregation-analysis

[11] Medical Author: William C. Shiel Jr., MD, FACP, FACR) Webster's New World medical dictionary. 2003. New York: Wiley.

[12] Molecular biology Glossary. https://www.genscript.com/molecular-biology-glossary/9184/concordance

[13] Research, Science and Therapy Committee of the American Academy of Periodontology. Informational paper: implications of genetic technology for the management of periodontal diseases. J Periodontol 2005;76(5):850-857.

[14] Kinane DF, Hart TC. Genes and gene polymorphisms associated with periodontal disease. Crit Rev Oral Biol Med 2003;14(6):430-449.

[15] Monaghan F, Corcos A. On the origins of the Mendelian laws. J Hered 1984; 75: 67-69.

[16] Kinane DF, Shiba H & Hart TC. The genetic basis of periodontitis. Perio 2000 2005; 39: 91-117.

[17] Singhal D, Mohan R, Krishna K, Kukreja BJ, Singh A. Genetics: applications in periodontal disease. TMU J Dent 2017; 4(4): 143-148.

[18] Hart TC. Genetic considerations of risk in human periodontal disease. Curr Opin Periodontol. 1994:3-11.

[19] Hodge P, Michalowicz B. Genetic predisposition to periodontitis in children and young adults. Periodontol 2000. 2001;26(1):113-134.

[20] Michalowicz BS, Diehl SR, Gunsolley JC, Sparks BS, Brooks CN, Koertge TE et al. Evidence of a substantial genetic basis for risk of adult periodontitis. J Periodontol 2000; 71(11): 1699-1707.

[21] Michalowicz BS, Wolff LF, Klump D, Hinrichs JE, Aeppli DM, Bouchard TJ Jr et al. Periodontal

bacteria in adult twins. J Periodontol 1999; 70(3): 263-273.

[22] Michalowicz BS, Aeppli D, Virag JG, Klump DG, Hinrichs JE, Segal NL et al. Periodontal findings in adult twins. J Periodontol 1991; 62(5): 293-299.

[23] Michalowicz BS, Aeppli DP, Kuba RK, Bereuter JE, Conry JP, Segal NL et al. A twin study of genetic variation in proportional radiographic alveolar bone height. J Dent Res 1991; 70(11): 1431-1435.

[24] Pihlstrom BL, Michalowicz BS, Johnson NW. Periodontal diseases. Lancet. 2005; 366(9499): 1809-1820.

[25] Schafer AS, Jepsen S, Loos BG. Periodontal genetics: a decade of genetic association studies mandates better study designs. J Clin Periodontol 2011; 38(2): 103-107.

[26] Boughman JA, Halloran SL, Roulston D, Schwartz S, Suzuki JB et al. An autosomal dominant form of periodontitis: its localization to chromosome 4 and linkage to dentinogenesis imperfecta. J Craniofac Genet Dev Biol 1986; 6: 341-350.

[27] Glazier AM, Nadeau JH, Aitman TJ. Finding genes that underlie complex traits. Science 2002: 298: 2345-2349.

[28] Townsend GC, Aldred MJ, Bartold PM. Genetic aspects of dental disorders. Aust Dent J 1998: 43: 269-286.

[29] Cantor RM, Rotter JI: Analysis of genetic data: methods and interpretation. In King RA, Rotter JI, Motulsky AG, editors: The genetic basis of common diseases, New York, 1992, Oxford University Press.

[30] Hodge SE. Linkage analysis versus association analysis: distinguishing between two models that explain disease marker associations. Am J Hum Genet 1993: 53: 367-384.

[31] Mc Carthy MI, Abecasis GR, Cardon LR, Goldstein DB, Little J, Ioannidis JP, Hirschhorn JN. Genome – wide association studies for complex traits. Consensus, Uncertainty and Challenges 2008; 9: 356-369.

[32] Melnick M, Shields ED, Bixler D. Periodontosis: A phenotypic and genetic analysis. Oral Surg Oral Med Oral Pathol 1976; 42: 32.

[33] Saxen L, Nevanlinna HR. Autosomal recessive inheritance of juvenile periodontitis: test of a hypothesis. Clin Genet 1984; 25: 332.

[34] Marazita ML, Burmeister JA, Gunsolley JC. Evidence for autosomal dominant inheritance and race specific heterogeneity in early onset periodontitis. J Periodontal 1994; 65: 623.

[35] Schenkein HA: Genetics of early onset periodontal diseases. In Genco R et al, editors: Molecular pathogenesis of periodontal disease, Washington, DC, 1994, American Society for Microbiology.

[36] Corey LA, Nance WE, Hofstede P. Self-reported periodontal disease in a Virginia twin population. J Periodontal 1992; 64: 1205.

[37] Li Y, Xu L, Hasturk H. Localized aggressive periodontitis is linked to chromosome 1q25. Hum Genet 2004; 114: 291.

[38] Tabeta K, Shimada Y, Tai H, Ishihara Y, Noguchi T, Soga Y, Yoshie H. Assessment of Chromosome 19 for Genetic Association in Severe Chronic Periodontitis. Journal of Periodontology 2009; 80(4): 663-671.

[39] Kornman KS, Di Giovine FS. Genetic variations in cytokine expression: A risk factor for severity of adult periodontitis. Ann Periodontol 1998; 3: 327.

[40] Gore EA, Sanders JJ, Pandey JP. Interleukin-1beta +3953 allele 2: association with disease status in adult periodontitis. J Clin Periodontol 1998; 25: 781.

[41] Kobayashi T. et al Relevance of immunoglobulin G Fc receptor polymorphism to recurrence of adult periodontitis in Japanese patients. Infect Immun 1997: 65: 3556-3560.

[42] Engebretson SP, Lamster IB, Herra-Abreu M. The influence of interleukin polymorphisms on expression of interleukin-1 and tumor necrosis factor a in periodontal tissue and gingival crevicular fluid. J Periodontol 1999; 70: 567.

[43] Galbraith GM, Steed RB, Sanders JJ. Tumor necrosis factor alpha production by oral leukocytes: influence of tumor necrosis factor genotype. J Periodontol 1998; 69: 428.

[44] Sofaer JA. Genetic approaches in the study of periodontal diseases. J Clin periodontal 1990; 17: 401.

[45] Terasaki PI, Kaslick RS, Westl TL. Low HL-A2 frequency and periodontitis. Tissue Antigens 1975; 5: 286.

[46] Katz J, Goultschin J, Benoliel R. Human leukocyte antigen DLR4: Positive association with rapidly progressing periodontitis. J Periodontol 1987; 58: 607.

[47] Babour S. Tobacco and smoking: environmental factors that modify the host response (immune system). Crit Rev Oral Biol Med. 1997;8:437-60.

[48] Aldred M.J. and Bartold P .M. Genetic disorders of the gingival and periodontium. Periodontol 2000 1998; 18:7-20.

[49] Kornman K.S., Crane A. and Wang H.Y. et al. The interleukin-1 genotype as a severity factor in adult periodontal disease. J Clin Periodontol 1997; 24:72-77.

[50] Genetics in Dentistry. GP Pal, NK Mahato, Jaypeepublications,2010

[51] Periodontics revisized, Shalu Bathla, Jaypee 20. Publications,2011

[52] Gandhi M, Kothiwale S. Association of periodontal diseases with genetic polymorphisms. International Journal of Genetic Engineering. 2012;2(3):19-27.

[53] Kinane DF, Hart TC. Genes and gene polymorphisms associated with periodontal disease. Critical Reviews in Oral Biology & Medicine. 2003 Nov;14(6):430-49.

[54] Greenstein G, Hart TC. A critical assessment of interleukin-1 (IL-1) genotyping when used in a genetic susceptibility test for severe chronic periodontitis. Journal of periodontology. 2002 Feb;73(2):231-47.

[55] Rogers et al. Do interleukin 1 polymorphisms predict the development of peridodonitis or the success of dental implants? J Periodont Res 2002; 37; 37-41.

[56] Huynh-Ba G., Lang N.P., Tonetti M.S. and Salvi G.E. The association of the composite IL-1 genotype with periodontitis progression and/or treatment outcomes: a systematic review. J Clin Periodontol 2007; 34(4):305-17.

[57] Nibali L, Ready DR, Parkar M, Brett PM, Wilson M, Tonetti MS, Griffiths GS. Gene polymorphisms and the prevalence of key periodontal pathogens. Journal of dental research. 2007 May;86(5):416-20.

[58] Vijayalakshmi R, Geetha A, Ramakrishnan T, Emmadi P. Genetic polymorphisms in periodontal diseases: an overview. Indian Journal of Dental Research. 2010 Oct 1;21(4):568.

[59] Schröder NW, Meister D, Wolff V, Christan C, Kaner D, Haban VA, Purucker P, Hermann C, Moter A, Göbel UB, Schumann RR. Chronic periodontal disease is associated with single-nucleotide polymorphisms of the human TLR-4 gene. Genes & Immunity. 2005 Aug;6(5):448-51.

[60] Kocher T, Sawaf H, Fanghänel J, Timm R, Meisel P. Association between bone loss in periodontal disease and polymorphism of N-acetyltransferase (NAT2). Journal of clinical periodontology. 2002 Jan;29(1):21-7.

[61] Newman,Takei, Klokkevold, Carranza. Carranza's Clinical Periodontology-11th ed. 2013.

[62] Wilton JMA, Griffiths GS, Curtis MA, Maiden MFJ, Gillett IR, Wilson DT, et al. Detection of high-risk groups and individuals for periodontal diseases. J Clin Periodontol 1988;15:339-46.

[63] Nualart Grollmus ZC, Morales Chávez MC, Silvestre Donat FJ. Periodontal disease associated to systemic genetic disorders. Medicina Oral, Patología Oral y Cirugía Bucal (Internet). 2007 May;12(3):211-5.

[64] Straub AM, Grahame R, Scully C, Tonetti MS. Severe periodontitis in Marfan's Syndrome: A Case Report. J Periodontol 2002;73:823-6.

[65] Castori M. Pain in Ehlers-Danlos syndromes: manifestations, therapeutic strategies and future perspectives. *Expert Opin Orphan Drugs*. 2016;4(11):1145-1158.(ehler)

[66] Perez LA, Al-Shammari KF, Giannobile WV, Wang H. Treatment of periodontal disease in a patient with Ehlers-Danlos Syndrome. A Case Report and literature review. J Periodontol 2002;73:564-70.

[67] Hakki SS, Aprikyan AAG, Yildirim S, Aydinbelge M, Gokalp A, Ucar C, et al. Periodontal status in two siblings with Severe Congenital Neutropenia: Diagnosis and Mutacional Analisis of the Cases. J Periodontol 2005;76:837-44.

[68] Saglam F, Atamer T, Oman U, Soidinç M, Kiraç K. Infantile Genetic Agranulocitosis (Kostmann Type). A Case Report. J Periodontol 1995; 66:808-10.

[69] Delcourt-Debruyne EMC, Boutigny HRA, Hildebrand HF. Features of severe periodontal disease in a teenager with Chediak-Higashi Syndrome. J Periodontol 2000;71:816-24.

[70] Izumi Y, Sugiyama S, Shinozuka O, Yamazaki T, Ohyama T, Ishikawa I. Defective neutrophil chemotaxis in Down's Syndrome patients and its relationship to periodontal destruction. J Periodontol 1989;60:238-41.

[71] Zaldivar-Chiapa RM, Arce-Mendoza AY, De La Rosa-Ramírez M, Caffesse RG, Solis-Soto JM. Evaluation of surgical and non-surgical periodontal therapies, and immunological status, of young Down's Síndrome patients. J Periodontol 2005;76:1061-5.

[72] Ullbro C, Brown A, Twetman S. Preventive periodontal regimen in Papillon-Lefevre Syndrome. Pediatr Dent 2005;27:226-32.

[73] Tsang P, Derkson G, Priddy R, Junker AK, Slots J, Larjava H. Severe periodontitis in a 5-years-old girl with hyperimmunoglobulin E Syndrome. Pediatr Dent 2005;27:68-73.

[74] Carlsson G, Wahlin YB, Johansson A, Olsson A, Eriksson T, Claesson R et al. Periodontal disease in patients from the original Kostmann family with severe congenital neutropenia. J Periodontol 2006;77:744-51.

[75] Borea G, Magi M, Mingarelli R, Zamboni C. The oral cavity in Down syndrome. J Pedodont 1990;14:139-40.

[76] Amanao A, Kishima T, Akiyama S, Nakagama I, Hamada S, Morisaki I. Relationship of periodontopathic bacteria with early-onset periodontitis in Down's Syndrome. J Periodontol 2001;72:368-73.

[77] Amanao A, Kishima T, Akiyama S, Nakagama I, Hamada S, Morisaki I. Periodontopathic bacteria in children with Down Syndrome. J Periodontol 2000;71:249-55.

[78] Periodontics revisited, Shalu Bathla, Jaypee publications,2011

[79] Hassell TM, Harris EL. Genetic influences in caries and periodontal diseases. Crit Rev Oral Biol Med 1995; 6(4): 319-342.

[80] Novak MJ, Novak KF. Early-onset periodontitis. Curr Opin Periodontol. 1996; 3: 45-58.

[81] Govindaraj P, Khan NA, Gopalakrishna P, Chandra RV, Vanniarajan A, Reddy AA et al. Mitochondrial dysfunction and genetic heterogeneity in chronic periodontitis. Mitochondrion. 2011; 11(3): 504-512.

[82] Taba Jr M, Jin Q, Sugai JV, Giannobile WV. Current concepts in periodontal bioengineering. Orthod Craniofac Res. 2005; 8(4): 292-302.

[83] Cirelli JA, Park CH, MacKool K, Taba Jr M, Lustig KH, Burstein H, et al. AAV2/1-TNFR:Fc gene delivery prevents periodontal disease progression. Gene Ther 2009; 16(3): 426- 436.

[84] Jin Q, Cirelli JA, Park CH, Sugai JV, Taba Jr M, Kostenuik PJ et al. RANKL inhibition through osteoprotegerin blocks bone loss in experimental periodontitis. J Periodontol 2007; 78(7): 1300-1308.

Chapter 6

The Role of Osteoporosis as a Systemic Risk Factor for Periodontal Disease

*Silvia Martu, Irina-Georgeta Sufaru,
Sorina-Mihaela Solomon, Ionut Luchian, Ioana Martu,
Liliana Pasarin, Dora-Maria Popescu,
Maria-Alexandra Martu and Monica-Silvia Tatarciuc*

Abstract

Periodontal disease is an infectious and inflammatory disease with a high incidence in the global population and an extremely complex etiopathogenesis. Osteoporosis is one of the systemic diseases that can affect the integrity of periodontal tissues. Osteoporosis, as a skeletal disease, causes a reduction in bone mass and microarchitectural changes in the bone. Discussions about the connection between the two diseases affecting the bone began in 1960, but, contrary to the high number of studies, discoveries are still being made regarding the pathophysiological mechanisms that link the two diseases. The chapter proposes a systematized description of data on the influence of osteoporotic disease on the periodontal structures, therapeutic methods to address the patient with periodontal disease and osteoporosis and data on the potential influence of conventional and adjunctive periodontal treatment on systemic parameters in patients with osteoporosis.

Keywords: periodontal disease, osteoporosis, inflammation, periodontal therapy

1. Introduction

In systemic diseases that can generate periodontal effects, it is worth mentioning osteoporosis as a separate entity in diseases of endocrine origin. Osteoporosis, as a skeletal disease, is characterized by reduced bone mass and micro-architectural changes in the bone that lead to bone fragility and an increased risk of fracture.

Bone tissues are dynamic, with healthy bone undergoing lifelong shaping and reshaping. Modelling is a process by which bone grows linearly in size in response to the stress applied to it. This involves bone neo-formation independent of a previous bone resorption, the skeleton being able to acquire new cortical shapes and thicknesses. On the other hand, remodelling is initiated by resorption and is followed by the formation of new bone tissue at the same resorption site. Bone remodelling repairs skeletal micro-destruction to preserve resistance and provides serum skeletal calcium for mineral homeostasis. Signals from mechanical stress are received by osteocytes and are transmitted to osteoclasts or osteoblasts or their precursors.

Bone resorption reflects the amount of osteoclast recruitment and death, as well as the rate of matrix degradation [1].

Hypothetical patterns linking the two conditions exist: it is assumed that reduced bone density in connection with osteoporosis may accelerate the resorption of alveolar bone caused by periodontitis, facilitating the invasion of pathogenic bacteria. This bacterial invasion affects normal bone homeostasis, increases osteoclastic activity, and reduces bone density both systemically and locally through both the direct effect of releasing toxins and the release of inflammatory mediators [2].

Since periodontal disease is a multifactorial condition, osteoporosis, although it may not be the cause of its onset, may be a factor in further exacerbation. Thus there is a greater predisposition to lose alveolar bone in subjects with osteoporosis, especially against the background of a pre-existing periodontal disease [3].

Oestrogen deficiency leads to the production of several cytokines produced by immune cells (monocytes and macrophages) and osteoblasts. When challenges arise from plaque biofilm products, bone resorption factors such as lipopolysaccharides, and toxins, the host's immune system produces several inflammatory cytokines that activate osteoclasts and cause bone resorption. The accumulation of bacterial plaque made up of periodontal bacteria seems to be necessary for a woman who is deficient in oestrogen to show changes such as loss of attachment and destruction of the alveolar bone.

The inflammatory response of the host to this biofilm starts the inflammatory cascade and can lead to a constant activation of proteinases and enzymes with the role of tissue degradation, leading to destruction of connective tissues, resorption of alveolar bone and finally bone loss, which explains the increased risk of periodontal damage in menopausal women [4].

Oestrogen deficiency-induced osteoporosis, characterized by an imbalance between bone formation and bone resorption, is caused by elevated inflammatory cytokines such as tumour necrosis factor α (TNFα), interleukin 1 (IL-1), IL-6 and gamma interferon (IFN-γ) [5]. Studies have shown that inflammatory cytokines increase osteoclast activity and activate bone resorption. Therefore, anti-resorptive therapy is widely used in the management of osteoporosis. This type of treatment, however, only prevents additional bone loss while barely stimulating bone formation and reversing bone loss. A number of studies have shown that elevated levels of inflammatory cytokines cause deficits in osteogenesis in postmenopausal osteoporosis and in inflammatory diseases such as arthritis and periodontitis [6].

2. Periodontal clinical and radiological status in patients with periodontal disease and osteoporosis

To date, most studies focused on the relationship between periodontal disease and osteoporosis have been performed in small groups, with limited control of bias factors, with significant variations in defining the parameters of periodontal disease and osteoporosis; there are also few longitudinal studies that establish a temporal relationship.

Decreased systemic bone density in patients with osteoporosis, including the jaw bones, may provide circumstances of increased susceptibility of these patients to periodontal damage.

Orthopantomography can be used as a complementary examination of the patient with osteoporosis and periodontal disease, to assess the width of the mandibular cortex, the cortical mandibular angle, the cortical index and the degree of resorption of the alveolar ridge. We conducted a study on a group of 41 subjects, whose aim was to evaluate radiological parameters on digital orthopantomography in patients with chronic periodontitis and osteoporosis, as well as to establish a correlation between them [7], bone mineral density and periodontal clinical parameters. For radiographic analysis we used digital orthopantomographs. The following determinations were made:

- Mandibular cortex thickness in the chin region (MCT)
- Panoramic mandibular index (PMI) - obtained by dividing the thickness of the mandibular cortex at the distance between the chin hole and the lower mandibular cortex
- Degree of resorption of the alveolar ridge (M/M ratio)
- Morphological classification of the lower mandibular cortex (C classes)

C1: normal bone cortex, with regular endo-osteal margin at both sides;

C2: moderately eroded bone cortex, with endo-osteal margin with semilunar defects;

C3: severely eroded bone cortex, with visibly porous endo-osteal margin.

The mean value of the plaque index was 1.21 ± 0.32. This index has been closely correlated with a C2 bone cortex class. A positive correlation was demonstrated between this index and the average loss of attachment. The mean value of the gingival index was 0.79 ± 0.21. This index was correlated with class C2 of bone cortex and with average loss of attachment. The mean value of the bleeding index was 2.3 ± 0.38, an index also correlated with class C2 of the bone cortex and loss of attachment. The mean value of the periodontal probe performed on all study participants was 4.72 ± 1.02 mm. There was no correlation between probing depth and bone resorption index [7].

The mean value of attachment loss was 4.35 ± 1.01 mm. There was a close positive correlation between the average loss of periodontal attachment and the C2 class of bone cortex. There was a negative correlation between mean attachment loss and bone resorption index. There was a link between the average loss of periodontal attachment and the plaque index, calculus index and gingival index [7].

A total of 58.7% of patients had 15–30 teeth remaining on the arches; 27.9% of the total number of examined patients had up to 15 remaining teeth and 13.4% of them - over 30 remaining teeth on the dental arches. A total of 36.5% of patients had loss of dental-periodontal units due to coronary dental lesions, 30.7% due to periodontal disease and 32.8% due to the association of carious lesions with periodontal disease. Only 3.8% of all patients had intact dental arches. Third molars were not considered in the calculation.

Using a threshold level of 3 mm for cortical thickness, only 2 patients had MCT <3 mm. We noticed an association between the T score value and MCT; low values of the T score were correlated with low values of cortical thickness ($p < 0.05$) [7].

We noticed that a decrease of MCT by 1 mm increases the risk of osteopenia/osteoporosis by 43%. The p value for MCT was statistically significant ($p = 0.033$). Moreover, when the morphology class is C2 or C3 (moderate and severe erosions), the age is increased and the MCT decreases to a statistically significant level ($p < 0.05$). A decrease of one millimetre of MCT increases the probability of moderately or severely eroded cortex by 96%. In terms of tooth loss, a one-unit increase in the number of missing teeth increases the probability of moderate or severe erosion by 6%.

Given that periodontal examination, along with performing oral radiographs are common procedures [8], the clinical significance for the observation of additional risk factors for osteoporosis is extremely high, and questions regarding skeletal status may arise. General condition of the patient.

An important result in this study is given by the close correlation between local factors and the loss of periodontal attachment and bone tissue. Moreover, the loss of attachment was closely related to the bone resorption index.

The oral cavity and jaws are examined radiologically more frequently than any other part of the human body. Orthopantomographic radiography can be a useful means of screening in the diagnosis of osteoporosis, providing valuable information on the quality of the maxillary bone.

The radiograph does not allow the visualization of the periodontal infection, nor the migration of the junction epithelium in the initial periodontal lesion. However, the radiographic image reflects the status of the mineralized structures of the periodontium. Thus, radiography is indispensable for assessing bone loss and for establishing residual value.

Clinical measurements by periodontal examination do not always fully and accurately reflect tissue loss, nor is radiography sufficient to establish a positive diagnosis. Radiography provides the image of two-dimensional bone changes, as well as abnormalities of radiopaque structures (carious, endodontic, reconstructive lesions). Radiographic images frequently used in periodontology are given by retro-dental-alveolar radiography, orthopantomography, as well as bite-wing radiography.

The panoramic x-ray represents a complex projection of the maxillary bones and dental arches, with multiple super-positions and distortions that can be exacerbated by image capture errors. Moreover, orthopantomography (OPT) illustrates numerous anatomical structures, in addition to the maxillary bones, which can represent interpretive challenges. In order to obtain a successful interpretation of panoramic radiographs, an understanding of the normal anatomy of the head and neck region and its radiologic aspects is absolutely mandatory.

Analysis of the density of the trabecular pattern of the maxillary bone, seen radiologically, showed that dense trabeculation is a strong indicator of increased mineral density, while thin trabeculation corresponds to low mineral density [9]. It is well known that in patients with osteoporosis the bone loss is not uniform and that the trabecular bone is earlier and more deeply affected than the cortical bone [10].

The mandible has a composition similar to the femoral neck [11], where fractures are mainly caused by a cortical loss rather than a trabecular bone. Given that the jaw consists mainly of trabecular bone, it is possible that the bone density measured at this level is more closely related to osteoporotic disease. However, the lack of fixed reference points in the upper jaw (such as the chin hole in the jaw) makes the assessment of standard points at this level a challenge.

Osteoporosis can be diagnosed by observing tooth loss, thinning of the lower mandibular cortex, and by changes in the morphology of the endo-osteal margin of the cortex and trabecular bone [12].

Mandibular bone mass correlates with systemic skeletal bone mass in numerous studies. Horner and Devlin reported a relationship between mandibular cortical thickness and mandibular bone density [12]. Cortical thickness at the gonial angle was determined by panoramic radiographs on a group of 180 patients; for patients aged 15 to 69 years, this was relatively constant; in subjects over 60 years of age, a decrease was observed, more significant for women than for men [13].

Devlin and Horner [12] reported that a cortical thickness of 3 mm is most appropriate as a threshold value for bone densitometry. White et al. [14] consider that this threshold value is more recommended to be 4 mm. Klemetti et al. [15] reported that the 4 mm threshold is optimal but not sufficient in itself for an optimal classification of subjects. In the present study we discovered values below 3 mm only on 3 radiographs; thus, we support the opinion of White et al. according to which, if panoramic radiographs are used, the threshold for cortical thickness is more appropriate at 4 mm [14].

As for quantitative computed tomography (QCT), it was first used to study the relationship between oral status and osteoporosis in 1989. Regardless of the technique used, the position of the sections and perspective should be documented by subsequent examinations to avoid the error of precision. The reported accuracy for QCT ranges from 1 to 3% for highly controlled settings and 4–5% for clinical settings [16]. Also, the cost of computed tomography is quite high, so it is not recommended only for a screening system in osteoporotic disease.

It has been demonstrated that mandibular cortex thickness can be a useful parameter to clinically assess metabolic bone loss and that a gonial thickness of less than 1 mm is an indicator of metabolic bone loss [12]. Dissemination of information on the prevention of osteoporosis produces a significant public effect for the implementation of appropriate ways to minimize the process of reducing bone mass.

3. The role of TNFα in patients with periodontal disease and osteoporosis

The main mechanism by which TNFα contributes to the evolution of osteoporosis is by disturbing the balance between bone resorption and bone formation [17]. Previously, TNFα blockade was considered to be an effective method to suppress and prevent bone resorption [18]. TNFα blockade significantly stimulated bone formation in mice.

We conducted a study of 46 postmenopausal female subjects in which we assessed the levels of TNFα in crevicular fluid and serum [19]. Subjects were divided into two groups: the Study Group - patients with osteoporosis and periodontal disease (n = 24) and the Control Group - patients with periodically healthy periodically disease (n = 22).

Probing depth (PD), bleeding on probing (BOP), and clinical attachment loss (CAL) had significantly higher values in the study group than in the control group ($p < 0.05$) [19]. We could not observe any significant differences in the values of the plate index between the groups.

All samples showed detectable levels of TNFα. Significantly high levels of TNFα were detected in both serum and GCF for the study group compared to the control group. Serum TNFα was positively correlated with BOP ($p < 0.01$). There were no significant correlations between probing depth, clinical attachment loss, plaque index, and TNFα levels. Serum TNFα levels were correlated with TNFα levels in crevicular fluid.

Maintaining the balance of proinflammatory and anti-inflammatory cytokines in the body is one of the manifestations of self-regulation [20]. Over the past decade, considerable evidence suggests that oestrogen prevents bone loss by blocking the production of proinflammatory cytokines, such as interleukin-1 (IL-1), IL-6, IL-10, tumour necrosis factor (TNF) α in the spinal cord and bone cells.

Cytokines are soluble proteins that can initiate, mediate, and control immune and inflammatory responses. It has been proposed that pro and anti-inflammatory cytokines contribute to various bone metabolic diseases, including periodontitis and postmenopausal osteoporosis [21]. Among pro-inflammators, TNFα has been reported to play a key role in periodontal bone destruction [22].

In our study we demonstrated significant differences in TNFα values between the osteoporosis group and the control group. It can be suggested that increased

TNFα values in GCF and serum contribute to the large number of B cells and T cells present in inflammatory periodontal tissues, increasing the destruction of periodontal tissue [19].

The fact that the values in the crevicular fluid were correlated with the serum values clearly indicates the influence that the systemic status generates on the local status (periodontal, in the case of the present study).

Periodontal tissue destruction is closely related to the release of inflammatory mediators, such as TNFα. These mediators are able to aggravate the inflammatory response. It has been shown that the severity of periodontal disease is associated with their concentration in the crevicular fluid.

Some subjects may have a more pronounced inflammatory response to bacterial aggression, a response that depends on the quality and quantity of the bacterial flora, as well as systemic factors (heredity, certain infectious/inflammatory diseases, osteoporosis, etc.).

Inflammatory cytokines can influence this delicate balance by promoting osteoclast differentiation and activation. Bone loss is thus attributed more to increased bone resorption than to reduced bone neo-formation, with osteoclasts being the main culprits.

4. The implications of the IL-1α and IL-1β cytokines in patients with periodontal disease and osteoporosis

IL-1α and IL-1β are biologically more or less equivalent pleiotropic factors that act locally and systemically. Only a few functional differences between the factors have been described; only IL-1β appears to be constitutively expressed in the brain. Interleukin-1 is a potent stimulator of bone resorption in vivo; IL-1β has been shown to be the most potent stimulator of bone resorption in vitro. The mechanism by which IL-1β stimulates resorption involves the expression of RANKL in osteoblasts and indirect stimulation of osteoclastogenesis and bone resorption [23].

There are also indications that osteoclasts express interleukin-1 receptor I, which is important for osteoclast activity and survival by activating the PI3K/AKT and ERK pathways, a MyD88-dependent response, but not on TRIF [24].

We conducted a study of 38 postmenopausal female subjects with the purpose to investigate differences in IL-1α and 1β levels in GCF in patients with chronic periodontitis, with or without associated chronic disease (in the present study - osteoporosis) [25].

IL-1α was the most prevalent cytokine found in GCF and was detected in all sites studied. We noticed significantly higher differences in interleukin levels for the study group (patients with osteoporosis) compared to systemically healthy patients ($p < 0.05$).

In order to establish the possible clinical relevance of these observations, a correlation analysis was performed between the clinical parameters and the total levels of cytokines in the test sites. Positive correlations were observed between IL-1α and 1β levels with PPD and CAL [25].

In periodontal inflammation, IL-1β is mainly expressed by macrophages and dendritic cells, but gingival fibroblasts, periodontal ligament cells, and osteoblasts can also secrete IL-1β. Elevated levels of IL-1β as well as IL-1α in gingival crevicular fluid have been reported by several groups [26]. There are many clinical studies showing the importance of IL-1β for inflammation and destruction in rheumatoid arthritis and osteoarthritis, associated with periodontal damage [27].

There are several reasons to believe that IL-1β could be an important mediator of the destruction of gingival connective tissue and periodontal ligament, as well as the resorption of alveolar bone. IL-1β is a potent stimulator of matrix metalloproteinase expression in fibroblasts and periodontal ligament cells [28].

The challenge in osteoimmunology is to determine the relative contribution of various components of the immune system to bone loss induced by ovariectomy and senile osteoporosis. These may also involve identical adjustment paths; however, in each system, there will be subtle differences in the net balance of local or systemic regulators, resulting in specific patterns of subsequent bone loss.

5. Influence of hormone replacement therapy on periodontal parameters in patients with osteoporosis

Hormone replacement therapy (HRT) represents an attractive method to counterbalance hormonal changes. The aim of HRT is not only to avoid climacteric signs and symptoms but also to protect the patients from cardiovascular disease and osteoporosis complications [29]. Having in mind that oestrogen deficit is an important risk factor for osteoporosis, it is of high importance to consider the role of oestrogen in the association between periodontal lesions and osteoporosis [30].

We proposed a comparative assessment of periodontal status in postmenopausal patients who were on hormone replacement therapy or not. The study was performed on a group of 23 female subjects, diagnosed with osteoporosis, aged between 50 and 62 years [30]. Subjects were divided into two groups. The first group, the study group, included patients undergoing hormone replacement therapy (n = 13); the control group included patients who did not follow this therapy (n = 10). The patients underwent periodontal clinical examination.

We noticed that the risk of tooth loss was similar for both groups but this risk shows a slight form of decrease with increasing treatment duration. Regarding the bleeding on probing, its value was approximately twice higher in patients without hormone replacement therapy, compared to the control group. The diagnosis of periodontal disease was higher in patients who did not receive replacement therapy than in those with HRT. In the group without hormone replacement therapy, we noticed more severe periodontal attachment losses than in the study group, with HRT. Moreover, the level of clinical attachment was proportional to the duration of hormone replacement therapy [30].

An important effect of low levels of oestrogen is the decrease in the inhibition of osteoclatogenesis, with a consequent increase in the activity of osteoclasts [31]. The result is a decrease in bone mass and bone resistance.

In vitro experiments indicate that neutrophil chemotaxis is reduced in the presence of low concentrations of estradiol. On the other hand, progesterone increases the chemotaxis of neutrophils, so any change in the balance of these hormones in plasma or gingival tissue can have a significant effect on neutrophil function in vivo [32].

Until recently, hormone replacement therapy was considered the only effective treatment recommended for the prevention of diseases associated with oestrogen deficiency [30]. After the publication of the Women's Health Initiative results in 2002 and 2004 [33], the use of HRT has become a complex debated issue. Women's Health Initiative and other data from dedicated studies suggested that the potential risks associated with HRT (increased risk of breast cancer and severe cardiovascular disease) are in direct relationship with the regimen administered, dose, mode of administration, age of the patient, associated disease, and duration of treatment [34]. Therefore, based on current data, the purpose, dose and regimen of HRT should be individualized, with a complex evaluation of each case [30].

Oestrogen has two key roles in bone health. First of all, the hormone is essential for the normal maturation of the bone and for ensuring the acquisition of minerals so as to reach an optimal bone mass. Second, oestrogen maintains bone mass throughout adulthood during remodelling processes. Oestrogen deficiency leads to a reduction in bone mass and damage to bone microarchitecture, the two being the main aspects of osteoporosis.

Oestrogen deficiency can cause bone loss by acting directly on bone cells that are involved in bone turnover and by decreasing the influence that oestrogen has on the intestines and kidneys that regulate extra-skeletal calcium levels.

Oestrogen deficiency contributes to the deterioration of bone microarchitecture and to the reduction of bone strength which is determined by bone geometry, cortical thickness, porosity, trabecular morphology. Bone remodelling results in the modification of major determinants of bone strength [35].

Oestrogen has been shown to stimulate osteoprotegerin (OPG) expression in human osteoblasts. The hormone can thus have an effect on bone metabolism through the surrounding soft tissue cells. Oestrogen has been shown to inhibit the formation of osteoclastic cells in cultures of fibroblasts in the periodontal ligaments and mononuclear cells in the peripheral blood. This inhibitory effect was not found in cultures with gingival fibroblasts. This observation suggests that they are not as sensitive to oestrogen without a clear biological mechanism. It is known that oestrogen exerts its effects through intercellular receptors; oestrogen receptor concentration is thus an important determinant of the cellular response to oestrogen.

The inhibitory effect of oestrogen on osteoclastic cell formation corresponds to previous research obtained either by osteoblast-induced osteoclast production or by bone marrow cells used as precursors. In addition, in vivo studies using ovariectomized mice have shown that oestrogen deficiency has induced the presence of a large number of osteoclasts in the periodontium. The data thus suggest that oestrogen plays an important role in modulating osteoclast formation.

Another important finding was the increased number of osteoclast-like cells in cultures with periodontal ligament fibroblasts. These observations suggest a difference in the interaction between different osteoblast populations and mononuclear cells in peripheral blood.

Subsequent analysis of molecules that may be involved in the oestrogen inhibitory effect involved the evaluation of mRNA expression of RANKL, OPG, and oestrogen receptors. No effect of oestrogen on the expression of these genes was found in any population of fibroblasts. The data suggest that the oestrogen inhibitory effect on osteoclastic cells can be mediated independently of OPG and RANKL, being mediated by other compounds such as TGF β, TNFα, IL-1, IL-6, IL-7 [30].

There are studies that have shown that the risk of edentulous ridges is lower in patients following HRT [36, 37]; it was observed that HRT reduced the risk of edentulousness by 6% for each year of HRT [38]. The patients with osteoporosis present a significant decrease in alveolar ridge height in edentulous areas and loss of alveolar ridge height is associated with osteoporosis and osteopenia [6]. We demonstrated a higher number of teeth present in patients with hormone replacement therapy [30]. However, teeth loss does not represent an ideal surrogate assessment for periodontal disease, as it can also be caused by carious lesions or traumatic events.

6. Effects of modulating inflammatory response therapy in patients with osteoporosis and chronic periodontitis

Mechanical removal of plaque and calculus from dental surfaces is considered the standard treatment for chronic periodontitis. Contrary to the spectacular evolution in the field of etiopathogenesis of periodontal disease, its treatment has changed very little, in principle. Scaling and root planing remain the "gold standard" of periodontitis treatment.

The importance of the host inflammatory response in periodontal pathogenesis presents the opportunity to explore new therapeutic strategies by means of modulating this response. Modulation therapy can be combined with conventional therapeutic methods to reduce the bacterial load.

To date, the only systemic therapy approved as a modulator of the response in periodontal disease is with sub-antimicrobial doses of doxycycline which inhibits the activity of matrix metalloproteinases (MMPs) (trade name: Periostat). Doxycycline in sub-antimicrobial doses inhibits MMP activity by synergistic mechanisms, independent of antibiotic properties. Primary studies have shown that the use of tetracycline predominantly inhibits MMPs in excess of periodontitis compared to constitutional MMPs. In vitro studies have shown that MMP-13 is more sensitive to tetracycline inhibitory concentrations than MMP-8 and MMP-1 (fibroblastic collagenase) is the least sensitive.

Doxycycline has been shown to be more effective than other tetracyclines in reducing collagenase activity in crevicular fluid in patients with chronic periodontitis [39]. Doxycycline has a lower inhibitory concentration than minocycline ($IC50 = 15$ IM compared to $IC50 = 190$IM) or tetracycline ($IC50 = 350$IM); thus, a lower dose of doxycycline than minocycline or tetracycline is required to reduce a certain level of collagenase by 50% [40]. Moreover, doxycycline is more effective in blocking the activity of neutrophil collagenase (MMP-8) than the activity of MMP-1 (fibroblastic collagenase), demonstrating that its use is a safe way to reduce pathological collagenase levels without affecting healthy tissues.

We conducted a study in a group of 26 subjects, with the purpose to analyse changes in periodontal clinical parameters that modulation therapy of the host response with sub-antimicrobial doses of doxycycline can exert in patients with periodontal disease and osteoporosis. Patients were randomly divided into two groups: the study group ($n = 17$), which underwent classical debridement therapy (scaling and root planing) plus sub-antimicrobial doses of doxycycline (20 mg twice daily) for 3 months, and control group ($n = 18$), which followed only classical debridement therapy [41].

We analysed the following periodontal parameters: probing depth, level of clinical attachment, PBI and PI index at baseline (pre-therapeutic), on the last day of medication, and 3 months after medication completion (6 months from baseline). The sites were grouped according to the probing depth in: group 1 - superficial (0-3 mm); group 2 - moderate (4-6 mm) and group 3 - deep (≥7 mm) [41].

In the present study, 30 patients were initially enrolled, but 4 of them failed to complete doxycycline therapy. Therefore, the study resulted in the use of two groups: the study group (13 subjects) and the control group (13 subjects). There was no statistically significant difference between groups at baseline in terms of probing depth. No significant differences were observed in the sites with an initial depth of 0–3 mm ($p > 0.05$). Significant reductions in probing depth were observed at sites with an initial depth of 4-6 mm and ≥ 7 mm ($p < 0.025$) [41].

Although the mean value of pocket reduction for sites with an initial depth of 4-6 mm and ≥ 7 mm was higher for the study group than for the control group

(1.80 mm versus 1.46 mm for moderate pockets and 3.38 mm versus of 2.57 mm for deep pockets), the difference did not reach the significance threshold ($p > 0.05$). Analysis of sites with an initial depth ≥ 7 mm showed that an increased percentage of sites was reduced by at least 3 mm following doxycycline administration (66.4%), compared to the group without modulation therapy (55.1%) at 3 months, without a statistically significant difference between groups ($p > 0.05$) [41].

However, at 6 months the percentage of sites with an improvement in depth ≥ 3 mm was significantly higher ($p = 0.011$) for the group with modulation therapy (73.4%) compared to the group that followed only classical therapy (49.7%) [41]. At baseline, there were no statistically significant differences in the level of clinical attachment in the sub-grouped sites by probing depth between the main study groups ($p > 0.05$). Sites with moderate depths and deep sites showed significant improvements in attachment level at 3 and 6 months, compared to baseline ($p < 0.025$). Sites with an initial depth of 0–3 mm did not show significant changes in attachment during the study period ($p > 0.05$) [41].

Sites with an initial depth of 0–3 mm in the control group (without doxycycline therapy) showed a slight decrease in attachment (−0.04 mm at 3 months, −0.03 mm at 6 months). On the other hand, the sites with the initial depth of 0-3 mm in the study group showed a slight gain of attachment (0.11 mm at 3 months, 0.14 mm at 6 months), but without significant differences between groups ($p > 0.05$).

Although the average attachment gains for sites with an initial depth of 4-6 mm and ≥ 7 mm was higher for the study group than for the control group (1.12 mm compared to 0.78 mm for sites with moderate depths; 2.15 mm compared to of 1.76 mm compared to the deep sites), the statistical analysis did not show a level of significance ($p > 0.05$) [41].

GDP and PI values showed significant improvements between baseline and re-evaluations at 3 and 6 months ($p < 0.025$). The reduction in GDP and IP was similar for both groups ($p > 0.05$).

Periodontal treatment, over time, has focused on reducing the bacterial load and disorganizing the biofilm by mechanical methods. However, recent research has led to a paradigm shift in the evolution of periodontal disease. Thus, it is known today that the lesions that appear at the level of superficial and deep periodontal tissues are a result of the activation of the host's immune-inflammatory defence mechanisms [42].

In addition to the classic periodontal therapy, scaling and root planing, which aims to disorganize the bacterial biofilm and reduce the inflammatory load, new adjunct methods have been postulated, with etiological therapeutic effect in the periodontopathic patient. Among them, the modulation therapy of the host's inflammatory response with pharmacological agents has acquired important dimensions, precisely because of its effectiveness. The success of such therapy is all the more important as it affects a systemically affected area.

Doxycycline has the ability to inhibit the activity of matrix metalloproteinases (MMPs), a capacity confirmed in numerous studies. Minocycline, doxycycline, and tetracycline inhibit collagenolytic activity, while non-tetracycline antibiotics have no effect on collagenase [40]. It was recognized in the mid-1980s that inhibition of collagenolysis by tetracyclines is a new therapeutic method in the management of periodontal disease.

The effects of doxycycline are, in addition to direct inhibition of active matrix metalloproteinases by cationic chelation and inhibition of oxidative activation of latent MMPs, and inhibition of the expression of inflammatory cytokines (IL-1, IL-6, TNFα) and PG-E2; seeks and inhibits the formation of oxygen-reactive species produced by neutrophils; protects the α1-proteinase inhibitor, thus indirectly reducing tissue proteinase activity; reduces osteoclastic activity and bone resorption; inhibits osteoclastic MMPs.

Doxycycline contributes to decreased conjunctival lysis by inhibiting pro-inflammatory mediators and cytokines (including IL-1 and TNFα) [43], as well as by increasing collagen production, osteoblast activity and bone formation [41]; this last aspect is of major importance especially for patients with osteoporosis, whose bone capital is affected.

A major concern with long-term administration of doxycycline has been associated with the development of antibiotic resistance. Indeed, when antimicrobial doses of tetracycline were used (250 mg daily, 2–7 years), up to 77% of patients' flora showed resistance to tetracycline [44]. Given this problem, sub-antimicrobial doses (20 mg doxycycline versus 50 or 100 mg) were prepared [41]. One of the preliminary experiments with this new formula clearly demonstrated that such doses (20 mg twice daily), administered 2 weeks, inhibited collagenase activity by 60–80% in gingival tissue in patients with chronic periodontitis [41]. Collagenase activity was significantly reduced in the crevicular fluid collected from these patients. Subsequent studies have indicated that this drug regimen can prevent the progression of periodontitis without the patient developing microorganisms resistant to doxycycline or other types of side effects [42].

The 3-month doxycycline regimen was well tolerated and no adverse reactions (gastrointestinal disorders, etc.) were reported. This may suggest that doxycycline modulation therapy is a safe approach in the long-term treatment of chronic periodontitis.

In the present study we observed improvements in clinical parameters (probing depth, level of clinical attachment, bleeding index, plaque index) both for the study group (with adjunctive modulation therapy) and for the control group (which followed only classical scaling-root planing therapy), improvements that were maintained throughout the study.

Caton et al. [45] established that reductions in probing depth of at least 3 mm represent relevant, clinically significant improvements. In the present study, the percentage of sites of great depth (≥7 mm) that showed reductions of at least 3 mm was significantly higher at 6 months for the group with modulation therapy. This result is of special importance, given that sites with such depth are candidates for surgical procedures. Therefore, it can be hypothesized that adjunctive doxycycline therapy may reduce the likelihood of surgical procedures as well as the discomfort caused by them [41].

We also demonstrated that the sites with relatively small depths (0-3 mm) in the study group showed a slight gain of attachment, while these sites in the control group showed a slight loss of attachment. This supports the efficacy of host response modulation therapy by administering sub-antimicrobial doses of doxycycline.

Studies are needed to evaluate the efficacy of very long-term sub-antimicrobial doses of doxycycline in periodontal therapy and in the prevention of loss of dental-periodontal units. The financial benefit derived from adjunctive therapy must also be evaluated (can this minimize costs by avoiding the need for periodontal surgery?).

It is suggested that doxycycline-based products be developed to support plasma concentrations for 24 hours by administering a single dose daily.

Given the increased variability of pathogenic pathways with a role in periodontal destruction (e.g., the cytokine group IL-1 is much more complex today), a more diverse range of host response modulators is also needed [46]. Moreover, most biological responses involve a variety of mechanisms; thus, blocking a single inflammatory pathway may not result in the desired result because receptor-mediated responses can be activated by alternative pathways. Therefore, a poly-pharmaceutical approach is needed to modify a number of different pathways associated with inflammation and tissue destruction.

Lipoxins are another group of compounds that can alter the inflammatory response in periodontal tissue. These mediators are released during the inflammatory response and have the effect of decreasing inflammation and modulating its disappearance. Lipoxins block the secretion of IL-1β from neutrophils and block the migration of neutrophils following exposure to *Porphyromonas gingivalis* [47].

Osteotrophic factors such as hormonal or endocrine-related (vitamin D3, parathyroid hormone), cytokines (IL-1, IL-6, IL-11 and IL-17), growth factors (TNFα, morphogenetic protein-2) and others molecules (PG-E2, LyT activator CD40 ligand and glucocorticoids) increase the expression of the RANKL gene in osteoblastic/stromal cells.

Sequentially, RANKL mediates the signal for ostoclastogenesis through RANK or preosteoclastic cells. Thus, the RANKL/RANK interaction is responsible for the differentiation and maturation of osteoclast precursor cells with osteoclast formation. Osteoprotegrin acts by binding to RANKL, inhibiting osteoclastic development.

In periodontal disease the first to investigate the role of RANKL in bone resorption was Teng [48]. It inoculated *Aggregatibacter actinomycetemcomitans* in mice lacking endogenous LyT and LyB and receiving human CD4 cells; Thus, CD4 + activation, RANKL stimulation and bone resorption were initiated, concluding that RANKL expression plays a significant role in bone destruction in periodontitis. Crotti et al. [49] observed a hyper-expression of RANKL in inflamed periodontal tissues, as well as an increased RANKL/osteoprotegrin ratio to healthy subjects.

There are numerous animal studies as well as preliminary human studies demonstrating inhibition of RANKL function by osteoprotegrin treatment, reducing the number of osteoclastic cells and, implicitly, bone resorption from periodontal disease. Of course, more in-depth studies are needed to certify the most effective therapeutic approach to this molecular interaction.

Fatty acids have been proposed to reduce chronic inflammation in arthritis patients by decreasing the release of LTB4 from neutrophils and IL-1 from monocytes. Local application of Omega-3 polyunsaturated fatty acids has been successful in patients with inflammatory diseases such as psoriasis, as well as in models with experimental periodontitis in animals. The mechanism of action is based on decreased leukocyte chemotaxis, expression of molecular adhesion and production of inflammatory cytokines. Offenbacher demonstrated the inhibition of PG-E2 production by eicosapentanoic or docosahexanoic acid administration, with effects similar to ibuprofen in patients with periodontal disease [50].

Vardar evaluated the use of omega-3 fatty acids in order to block arachidonic acid cascade in mice with experimentally induced periodontal disease [51]. This would inhibit the production of cyclooxygenase-derived prostanoids and lipo-oxygenase-derived leukotrienes. The authors relied on two aspects: leukotriene B4 (mediator of arachidonic acid) plays an important role in bone resorption and inhibition of COX with NSAIDs would cause the accumulation of arachidonic acid that is metabolized by lipo-oxygenase, causing continuous bone loss. The authors also administered a combination of omega-3 fatty acids with celecoxib, seeking a synergistic anti-inflammatory effect. Combination therapy resulted in significant decreases in prostaglandin, leukotriene B4 and PAF levels; no effect on bone lysis was observed (this may be due to the short evaluation period).

Elkhouli published the results of a study of 40 patients with at least one grade II furcation defect; patients were divided into two groups: the first group performed allografting, which was associated with therapy with omega-3 polyunsaturated fatty acids and low-dose aspirin; in the second group (control) only allografting was performed, following a placebo adjunctive therapy. At 3 and 6 months, the clinical parameters (plaque index, gingival index, bleeding index, probing depth, level of clinical attachment) were evaluated, as well as biochemical markers in the crevicular fluid (IL-1b and IL-10) [52]. The results were very good for the test group compared to the control group (reduction of probing depth, gain of clinical attachment, significant modulating effect for IL-1b and IL-10 levels).

There are proven clinical results regarding monounsaturated fatty acid substitution; they influence blood pressure, clotting, endothelial activation, inflammation and thermogenic capacity in cardiac patients, they prevent obesity and other metabolic diseases.

Hasturk demonstrated in a study in rabbits with experimentally induced periodontitis with *Porphyromonas gingivalis* that topical application of the tetradecanol-1 complex (1-TDC: mixture of esterified monounsaturated fatty acids) causes an inhibitory effect on the inflammatory cascade of the host response [53].

Further studies are needed to evaluate the impact of this modulation therapy in patients with periodontal disease and osteoporosis at the molecular level (by examination of the crevicular fluid), on pro-inflammatory cytokines, and at the systemic level, by assessing bone mineral density (correlation with pre- and post-therapeutic T score).

7. Conclusions and perspectives

Chronic periodontitis and osteoporosis are two chronic diseases, with inflammatory etiopathogenesis, whose statistical characteristics are constantly growing worldwide. Studies focused on the association of these diseases in the same subjects are few and with discordant results. These may be due to the variability of the inclusion/exclusion criteria, the research methodology, as well as the small groups of subjects included.

The research supports the role that a routine operation performed in the dental office - panoramic radiography - could play in detecting undiagnosed cases of osteoporosis, given the local changes that occur in such patients. Signs of periodontal tissue destruction are also reflected radiologically, where the thickness of the mandibular cortex and the morphological appearance of the cortex (presence of erosions) have been shown to be closely correlated with the value of the densitometric T Score. Therefore, orthopantomography, a common procedure in the dental office, could be an effective and less expensive method of screening for osteoporosis, with a significant role for the dentist in this procedure.

Despite advances in research methodology and laboratory tests, in order to identify the factors associated with chronic periodontal disease, it is still unclear how to predict the progression of periodontal disease. Extensive research has been done in the area of host biochemical response markers in periodontal disease. It is unlikely that a unitary biomarker will be able to meet the criteria for estimating future destruction from periodontal disease.

Patients with periodontal disease with osteoporosis had higher levels of TNFα, IL-1α, IL-1β, IL-6 and RANKL in the crevicular fluid, compared to systemically healthy patients. Also, cytokine values were positively correlated with periodontal parameters. Therefore, it can be stated that these patients are prone to excessive production of this type of cytokine which also activates B cells and promotes B cell activity in periodontal inflammatory sites, aggravating the evolution of periodontal disease.

The conventional systemic hormone replacement therapy was associated with lower indices of gingival inflammation, such as a reduced gingival bleeding index in subjects who followed hormone replacement therapy when compared to the subjects without HRT [30]. The risk of tooth loss was reduced in the group with HRT, when compared to patients without HRT and, more importantly, the number of present teeth is directly proportional to the duration of the substitution therapy [30]. The diagnosis of periodontal disease was more common in patients without hormone replacement therapy compared to those with HRT. We can conclude that HRT generates a positive effect on periodontal tissues, an effect that is all the better highlighted as hormone replacement therapy has a longer duration; still, this benefit needs to be carefully assessed and compared to the potential risks of such therapy [30]. These aspects bring in a new sphere the ways of complex and interdisciplinary therapeutic approach of patients with osteoporosis and chronic periodontitis.

We also proposed a unique analysis in the context of the association of the two diseases - periodontal disease and osteoporosis - of the effects generated by a deputy form of periodontal therapy, extremely topical, that of modulation therapy by chemotherapeutic agents of the host's inflammatory response. We demonstrated in the study that adjunctive therapy with sub-antimicrobial doses of doxycycline (administration of 20 mg twice daily, 3 months), in combination with classical therapy, generated significant clinical improvements in patients with periodontal disease and osteoporosis - maintained during the study and that could pre-meet the need for surgery. We also demonstrated that sites with relatively small depths (0-3 mm) in the modulation therapy group showed a slight gain in attachment, while these sites in the control group showed a slight loss of attachment. This supports the efficacy of host response modulation therapy by administering sub-antimicrobial doses of doxycycline. Taken together, the data presented should inspire further research, providing epigenetic responses in periodontics, and using this information to develop future therapies.

The set of studies carried out supports in a complex way the importance of the bidirectionality of the periodontal disease - osteoporosis relationship, offering new information and protocols to approach patients, with certain value both for the medical community and, especially, for the entity that is at the centre of its concern - the patient per se.

Studies have shed new light on the link between periodontal disease (particularly in its chronic form) and osteoporosis. The data obtained show observations of a clinical and paraclinical nature, which aim to expand the knowledge related to this complex association, with practical applicability, which supports the concept of interdisciplinary approach to the patient.

Periodontal tissue damage, clinically detectable by measurements of periodontal parameters (probing depth, loss of clinical attachment, probing bleeding), is more severe in patients with osteoporosis than in systemically healthy patients. Research has shown that osteoporosis systemically creates favourable circumstances for the evolution of periodontal disease, but it is also significantly associated with local determinants and factors.

Conflict of interest

The authors declare no conflict of interest.

Author details

Silvia Martu[1], Irina-Georgeta Sufaru[1*], Sorina-Mihaela Solomon[1], Ionut Luchian[1], Ioana Martu[1], Liliana Pasarin[1], Dora-Maria Popescu[2], Maria-Alexandra Martu[1] and Monica-Silvia Tatarciuc[1]

1 "Grigore T. Popa" UMPh, Iasi, Romania

2 UMPh, Craiova, Romania

*Address all correspondence to: irina_ursarescu@yahoo.com

References

[1] Friedlander AH. The physiology, medical management and oral implication of menopause. Journal of American Dental Association. 2002;133:73-81. DOI: https://doi.org/10.14219/jada.archive.2002.0025

[2] Guiglia R, Di-Fede O, Lo-Russo L Sprini D, Rini GB, Campis G. Osteoporosis, jawbones and periodontal disease. Medicina Oral Patologia Oral Cirugia Bucal. 2013;18:93-99. DOI: 10.4317/medoral.18298

[3] Esfahanian V, Shamami MS, Shamami MS. Relationship between osteoporosis and periodontal disease: Review of the literature. Journal of Dentistry (Teheran). 2012;9:256-264. PMCID: PMC3536461

[4] Buencamino M, Palomo L, Thacker HL. How menopause affects oral health, and what we can do about it. Cleveland Clinical Journal of Medicine. 2009;768:467-475. DOI: 10.3949/ccjm.76a.08095

[5] Brennan RM, Genco RJ, Hovey KM, Trevisan M, Wactawski-Wende J. Clinical attachment loss, systemic bone density, and subgingival calculus in postmenopausal women. Journal of Periodontology. 2007;78:2104-2111. DOI: 10.1902/jop.2007.070155

[6] Tezal M, Wactawski-Wende J, Grossi SG, Ho AW, Dunford R, Genco RJ. The relationship between bone mineral density and periodontitis in postmenopausal women. Journal of Periodontology. 2000;71:1492-1498. DOI: 10.1902/jop.2000.71.9.1492

[7] Ursarescu I, Solomon S, Potarnichie O, Pasarin L, Martu I, Luchian I, martu S. The evaluation of clinical and imagistic parameters on osteoporosis patients. Romanian Journal of Oral Rehabilitation. 2012;4:53-57.

[8] Marques MR, Da Silva MAD, Barros SP. Periodontal Disease and Osteoporosis Association and Mechanisms: a Review of the Literature. Brasilian Journal of Oral Science. 2003;2:137-140. DOI: 10.1016/j.archoralbio.2004.08.014

[9] Jonasson G, Bankvall G, Kiliaridis S. Estimation of skeletal bone mineral density by means of the trabecular pattern of the alveolar bone, its interdental thickness, and the bone mass of the mandible. Oral Surgery Oral Medicine Oral Pathology Oral Radiology and Endodontology. 2001;92:346-352. DOI: 10.1067/moe.2001.116494

[10] Khosla S. Pathogenesis of age-related bone loss in humans. The Journals of Gerontology Series A Biological Sciences and Medical Sciences. 2013;68:1226-1235. DOI: 10.1093/gerona/gls163

[11] Devlin H, Whelton C. Can mandibular bone resorption predict hip fracture in elderly women? A systematic review of diagnostic test accuracy. Gerodontology. 2013;32:163-168. DOI: https://doi.org/10.1111/ger.12077

[12] Devlin H, Horner K. Mandibular radiomorphometric indices in the diagnosis of reduced skeletal bone mineral density. Osteoporosis International. 2002;13:373-378. DOI: 10.1007/s001980200042

[13] Bras J, van Ooij CP, Abraham-Inpijn L, Kusen GJ, Wilmink JM. Radiographic interpretation of the mandibular angular cortex: A diagnostic tool in metabolic bone loss. Part I. Normal state. Oral Surgery Oral Medicine Oral Pathology. 1982;53:541-545. DOI: 10.1016/0030-4220(82)90473-x

[14] White SC, Taguchi A, Kao D, Wu S, Service SK. Clinical and panoramic

predictors of femur bone mineral density. Osteoporosis International. 2005;16:339-346. DOI: 10.1007/s00198-004-1692-4

[15] Klemetti E, Kalmakov S, Kroger H. Pantomography in assessment of the osteoporosis risk group. Scandinavian Journal of Dental Research. 1994;102:68-72. DOI: 10.1111/j.1600-0722.1994.tb01156.x

[16] Lang P, Steiger P, Faulkner K, Gluer C, Genant HK. Osteoporosis. Current techniques and recent developments in quantitative bone densitometry. Radiologic Clinics of North America. 1991;29:49-76. PMID: 1985329

[17] Nanes MS. Tumor necrosis factor-alpha: molecular and cellular mechanisms in skeletal pathology. Gene. 2003;321:1-15. DOI: 10.1016/s0378-1119(03)00841-2

[18] Cenci S, Weitzmann MN, Roggia C, Namba N, Novack D, Woodring J, Pacifici R. Estrogen deficiency induces bone loss by enhancing T-cell production of TNF-alpha. The Journal of Clinical Investigation. 2000;106:1229-1237. DOI: 10.1172/JCI11066

[19] Ursarescu I, Pasarin L, Solomon S, Boatca RM, Martu A, Moise G, Martu S. The assessment of serum and GCF proinflammatory cytokines levels in patients with osteoporosis and periodontal disease. Romanian Journal of Oral Rehabilitation. 2014:6:45-50.

[20] Garlet GP, Martins WJ, Fonseca BA, Ferreira BR, Silva JS. Matrix metalloproteinases, their physiological inhibitors and osteoclast factors are differentially regulated by the cytokine profile in human periodontal disease. Journal of Clinical Periodontology. 2004;31:671-679. DOI: 10.1111/j.1600-051X.2004.00545.x

[21] Miyazaki T, Matsunaga T, Miyazaki S, Hokari S, Komoda T. Changes in receptor activator of nuclear factor kappaB, and its ligand, osteoprotegerin, bone-type alkaline phosphatase, and tartrate-resistant acid phosphatase in ovariectomized rats. Journal of Cellular Biochemistry. 2004;93:503-512. DOI: 10.1002/jcb.20201

[22] Graves D. Cytokines that promote periodontal tissue destruction. Journal of Periodontology. 2008;79:1585-1591. DOI: 10.1902/jop.2008.080183

[23] Lorenzo J, Horowitz M, Choi Y. Osteoimmunology: Interactions of the bone and immune system. Endocrine Reviews. 2008;29:403-440. DOI: 10.1210/er.2007-0038

[24] Sato N, Takahashi N, Suda K, Nakamura M, Yamaki M, Ninomiya T, Kobayashi Y, Takada H, Shibata K, Tamamoto M, Takeda K, Akira S, Noguchi T, Udagawa N. MyD88 but not TRIF is essential for osteoclastogenesis induced by lipopolysaccharide, diacyl lipopeptide, and IL-1a. Journal of Experimental Medicine. 2004;200:601-611. DOI: https://doi.org/10.1902/jop.2008.080183

[25] Ursarescu IG, Paval D, Solomon SM, Pasarin L, Boatca M, Nicolaiciuc O, Nitescu DC, Martu S. Study regarding the IL1-A and IL1-B levels in gingival crevicular fluid in patients with chronic periodontitis and osteoporosis. Romanian Journal of Oral Rehabilitation. 2016:8:97-102.

[26] Holmlund A, Hanstrom L, Lerner UH. Bone resorbing activity and cytokine levels in gingival crevicular fluid before and after treatment of periodontal disease. Journal of Clinical Periodontology 2004; 31: 475-482. DOI: 10.1111/j.1600-051X.2004.00504.x

[27] Daheshia M, Yao JQ. The interleukin-1a pathway in the

pathogenesis of osteoarthritis. The Journal of Rheumatology. 2008;35:2306-2312. DOI: 10.3899/jrheum.080346

[28] Cox SW, Eley BM, Kiili M, Asikainen A, Tervahartiala T, Sorsa T. Collagen degradation by interleukin-1a-stimulated gingival fibroblasts is accompanied by release and activation of multiple matrix metalloproteinases and cysteine proteinases. Oral Diseases 2006;12:34-40. DOI: 10.1111/j.1601-0825.2005.01153.x

[29] Grodstein F, Stampfer R. The epidemiology of coronary heart disease and estrogen replacement in postmenopausal women. Progress in Cardiovascular Diseases. 1995;38:199-121. DOI: https://doi.org/10.1016/S0033-0620(95)80012-3

[30] Laza GM, Sufaru IG, Martu MA, Anton D, Mocanu R, Pasarin L, Surlin P. The role of hormone replacement therapy in patients with osteoporosis and periodontal disease. Romanian Journal of Medical and Dental Education. 2020:9:6-12.

[31] Teitelbaum SL. Bone resorption by osteoclasts. Science. 2000;289:1504-1508. DOI: 10.1126/science.289.5484.1504

[32] Knight ET, Liu J, Seymour GJ, Faggion CM Jr, Cullinan MP. Risk factors that may modify the innate and adaptive immune response in periodontal diseases. Periodontology 2000. 2016;71:22-51. DOI: 10.1111/prd.12110

[33] Anderson GL, Limacher M, Assaf AR, Bassford T, Beresford SAA, Black H, Bonds D, Brunner R, Brzyski R, Caan B, Chlebowski R, Curb D, Gass M, Hays J, Heiss G, Hendrix S, Howard BV, Hsia J, Hubbell A, Jackson R, Johnson KC, Judd H, Morley Kotchen J, Kuller L, LaCroix AZ, Lane D, Langer RD, Lasser N, Lewis CE, Manson J, Margolis K, Ockene J, O'Sullivan MJ, Phillips L, Prentice RL, Ritenbaugh C, Robbins J, Rossouw JE, Sarto G, Stefanick ML, Van Horn L, Wactawski-Wende J, Wallace R, Wassertheil-Smoller S, Women's Health Initiative Steering Committee. Effects of conjugated equine estrogen in postmenopausal women with hysterectomy: the Women's Health Initiative randomized controlled trial. Journal of American Medical Association. 2004;291:1701-1712. DOI: 10.1001/jama.291.14.1701

[34] Santen RJ, Allred DC, Ardoin SP, Archer DF, Boyd N, Braunstein GD, Burger HG, Colditz GA, Davis SR, Gambacciani M, Gower BA, Henderson VW, Jarjour WN, Karas RH, Kleerekoper M, Lobo RA, Manson JE, Marsden J, Martin KA, Martin L, Pinkerton JW, Rubinow DR, Teede H, Thiboutot DM, Utian WH. Postmenopausal hormone therapy: an Endocrine Society scientific statement. The Journal of Clinical Endocrinology & Metabolism. 2010;95:s1–s66. DOI: https://doi.org/10.1210/jc.2009-2509

[35] Reid DM. The Handbook of Osteoporosis. New York; Springer; 2011. p. 19-22. DOI: 10.1007/978-1-908517-10-4

[36] Meisel P, Reifenberger J, Haase R, Nauck M, Bandt C, Kocher T. Women are periodontally healthier than men, but why don't they have more teeth than men? Menopause. 2008;15:270-275. DOI: 10.1097/gme.0b013e31811ece0a

[37] Taguchi A, Sanada M, Suei Y, Ohtsuka M, Nakamoto T, Lee K, Tsuda M, Ohama K, Tanimoto K, Bollen AM. Effect of estrogen use on tooth retention, oral bone height, and oral bone porosity in Japanese postmenopausal women. Menopause. 2004;11:556-562. DOI: 10.1097/01.gme.0000113845.74462.bf

[38] Krall EA, Dawson-Hughes B, Hannan MT, Wilson PWF, Kiel DP. Postmenopausal estrogen replacement

and tooth retention. The American Journal of Medicine. 1997;102:536-542. DOI: https://doi.org/10.1016/S0002-9343(97)00045-4

[39] Golub LM, Wolff M, Lee HM, McNamara TF, Ramamurthy NS, Zambon J, Ciancio S. Further evidence that tetracyclines inhibit collagenase activity in human crevicular fluid and from other mammalian sources. Journal of Periodontal Research. 1985;20:12-23. DOI: 10.1111/j.1600-0765.1985.tb00405.x

[40] Golub LM, Wolff M, Roberts S, Lee HM, Leung M, Payonk GS. Treating periodontal diseases by blocking tissue-destructive enzymes. The Journal of American Dental Association. 1994;125:163-169. DOI: 10.14219/jada.archive.1994.0261

[41] Ursarescu I, Solomon S, Rudnic I, Potarnichie O, Martu S. Evaluation of the effects of hormonal substitution therapy upon the periodontal status in female patients during pre-and post-menopause. International Journal of Medical Dentistry. 2012:16:300-304.

[42] Offenbacher S, Barros SP, Beck JD. Rethinking periodontal inflammation. Journal of Periodontology. 2008;79:1577-1584. DOI: 10.1902/jop.2008.080220

[43] Milano S, Arcoleo F, D'Agostino P, Cillari E. Intraperitoneal injection of tetracyclines protects mice from lethal endotoxemia downregulating inducible nitric oxide synthase in various organs and cytokine and nitrate secretion in blood. Antimicrobial Agents and Chemotherapy. 1997;41:117-121. PMID: 8980766

[44] Kornman KS, Karl EH. The effect of long-term low-dose tetracycline therapy on the subgingival microflora in refractory adult periodontitis. Journal of Periodontology. 1982;53: 604-610. DOI: 10.1902/jop.1982.53.10.604

[45] Caton JG, Ciancio SG, Blieden TM, Bradshaw M, Crout RJ, Hefti AF, Massaro JM, Polson AM, Thomas J, Walker C. Treatment with subantimicrobial dose doxycycline improves the efficacy of scaling and root planing in patients with adult periodontitis. Journal of Periodontology. 2000;71:521-532. DOI: 10.1034/j.1600-051x.2001.280810.x

[46] Barksby HE, Lea SR, Preshaw PM, Taylor JJ. The expanding family of interleukin-1 cytokines and their role in destructive inflammatory disorders. Clinical & Experimental Immunology. 2007;149:217-225. DOI: 10.1111/j.1365-2249.2007.03441.x

[47] Pouliot M, Clish CB, Petasis NA, Van Dyke TE, Serhan CN. Lipoxin A(4) analogues inhibit leukocyte recruitment to Porphyromonas gingivalis: a role for cyclooxygenase-2 and lipoxins in periodontal disease. Biochemistry. 2000;39:4761-4768. DOI: 10.1021/bi992551b

[48] Teng YTA. Mixed periodontal Th1-Th2 cytokine profile in Actinobacillus actinomycetemcomitans-specific osteoprotegerin Ligand (or RANK-L)- mediated alveolar bone destruction in vivo. Infection and Immunity. 2002;70:5269-5273. DOI: 10.1128/IAI.70.9.5269-5273.2002

[49] Crotti T, Smith MD, Hirsch R, Soukoulis S, Weedon H, Capone M, Ahersn MJ, Haynes D. Receptor activator NF kappaB ligand (RANKL) and osteoprotegerin (OPG) protein expression in periodontitis. Journal of Periodontal Research. 2003;38:380-387. DOI: 10.1034/j.1600-0765.2003.00615.x

[50] Offenbacher S, Heasman PA, Collins JG. Modulation of host PGE2 secretion as a determinant of periodontal disease expression. Journal of Periodontology. 1993;64:432-444. DOI: 10.1902/jop.1993.64.5s.432

[51] Vardar S, Baylas H, Huseyinov A. Effects of selective cyclooxygenase-2 inhibition on gingival tissue levels of prostaglandin E2 and prostaglandin F2a and clinical parameters of chronic periodontitis. Journal of Periodontology. 2003;74:57-63. DOI: 10.1902/jop.2003.74.1.57

[52] Elkhouli AM. The efficacy of host response modulation therapy (omega-3 plus low-dose aspirin) as an adjunctive treatment of chronic periodontitis (clinical and biochemical study). Journal of Periodontal Research. 2011;46:261-268. DOI: 10.1111/j.1600-0765.2010.01336.x

[53] Hasturk H, Kantarci A, Ohira T, Arita M, Ebrahimi N, Chiang N, Petasis NA, Levy BD, Serhan CN, van Dyke TE. RvE1 protects from local inflammation and osteoclastmediated bone destruction in periodontitis. The FASEB Journal. 2006;20:401-403. DOI: 10.1096/fj.05-4724fje

Chapter 7

The Complex Relationship of Periodontal Disease and Rheumatoid Arthritis

Maria-Alexandra Martu, Elena Rezus, Diana Tatarciuc, Ionut Luchian, Irina-Georgeta Sufaru, George-Alexandru Maftei, Dorin Gheorghe, Liliana Pasarin, Sorina Mihaela Solomon and Liliana Georgeta Foia

Abstract

The relationship between periodontitis and systemic diseases is an important part of clinical periodontal research, which has been growing steadily. Even though the etiologies of periodontal disease and rheumatoid arthritis (RA) differ, these pathologies have many common features, both being multifactorial diseases characterized by localized chronic inflammatory reactions, which are fuelled by an analogous set of cytokines (among many, the most prominent being Tumour Necrosis Factor (TNF), Interleukin (IL) 6 and 17), leading to high systemic circulating concentrations of inflammatory markers such as C-reactive protein (CRP). It was not until the discovery of peptidylarginine deiminase (PAD) mediated citrullination of proteins by *Porphyromonas gingivalis* that the link between the two diseases was purely speculative. This citrullination initiates a series of events which culminate in the production of anti-citrullinated protein antibodies (ACPA) and, finally, in the clinical manifestation of rheumatoid arthritis. Another common denominator is the bone destruction caused by proinflammatory cytokines secreted by T 17 helper cells (TH17) which is the pathological hallmark of both diseases. Other notable common areas are shared risk factors such as environmental and genetic risk factors. Regarding treatment, neither pathologies have a definitive cure, however, several strategies are employed, some of which are common, such as diet and lifestyle changes, and immunomodulating medication applied locally or systemically.

Keywords: periodontal disease, rheumatoid arthritis, cytokines, DMARDS, treatment, microorganisms

1. Introduction

The relationship between periodontitis and systemic disease is an important part of clinical periodontal research, which has been growing steadily since the late 1980s. Monsarrat et al., in 2016 stated that approximately a third of all recent periodontal studies address this issue [1]. Moreover, in the same year Loos published the results of a study, accrediting the fact that a total of 57 different systemic diseases are being investigated for possible links [2].

This relationship is often described as "bidirectional", but the design of many epidemiological observational studies does not allow the relationship to be firmly established and, implicitly, any identified associations will be bidirectional until clarifying data appear. At present, there is no full understanding of the importance of the multiple associations reported and especially whether they play a causal role.

Although having different etiologies, periodontal disease (PD) and rheumatoid arthritis (RA) have many common features, both being multifactorial diseases characterized by localized chronic inflammatory reactions, which are fed by an analogous set of cytokines (Tumour Necrosis Factor (TNF)-α, Interleukins (IL) 6 and 17), leading to high concentrations of inflammatory markers such as circulating C-reactive protein (CRP) [3]. In addition, bone destruction caused by proinflammatory cytokines secreted by helper T cells (TH17) is the pathological hallmark of both diseases. Furthermore, periodontitis and RA have certain risk factors in common such as environmental and genetic [4].

Rheumatoid arthritis is a chronic, autoimmune systemic inflammatory disease, characterized by an arthropathy with chronic, progressive, deforming and destructive evolution, having a major disabling character and multiple systemic manifestations that determine an important premature mortality. It affects 0.5-1.0% of the world's population, the cause however is still unclear [5]; having said all this, it is thought to be triggered by a combination of genetic and environmental factors that lead to the degradation of immune tolerance at the interface with mucosal surfaces, specifically in the lungs, intestines, and periodontium [6]. The effect is the triggering of the autoimmune response characterized by the production of rheumatoid factor (FR) and ACPA (anticitrullinated protein antibodies). Binding of ACPA to citrullinated epitopes in joints and the formation of immune complexes containing rheumatoid factor helps to form a vicious circle of tissue damage involving the activation of synovial macrophages and dendritic cells, and the release of proinflammatory cytokines and enzymes that lead to tissue degradation. At the same time, peptidilarginine deiminases (PAD) released by neutrophils during necrosis or during the production of extracellular traps citrullinate the proteins in the joints, resulting in a continuous local immune response that is self-sustaining [7].

Until a few years ago, despite these common features, it was difficult, if not impossible, to establish a potential causal link between the two diseases. The discovery and characterization of an enzyme uniquely expressed by the major pathogen in periodontal disease *Porphyromonas gingivalis*, namely peptidilarginine deiminase (called PPAD to distinguish this bacterial enzyme from human peptidilarginine deiminase - PAD), was the basis for the hypothesis that protein citrullination mediated by PPAD originating from inflamed periodontal sites may initiate a series of events that culminate in the production of anti-citrulline protein antibodies (ACPA) and ultimately in the clinical manifestation of RA [8].

The diagnosis of RA has been revolutionized by the discovery of ACPA, disease-specific antibodies that are present in approximately 70% of patients with this pathology. These are strictly correlated with the severity of the disease and with major risk factors, genetic and environmental, suggesting a pathogenic involvement. They are also detectable in the bloodstream 10 years before the onset of clinical symptoms, suggesting that the initial loss of immune tolerance to citrullinate proteins is most likely a consequence of an inflammatory event that occurs outside the joint [9].

However, most proteins in the human body undergo certain post-translational changes, starting with proteolytic modifications, glycosylation processes or lipid changes, to modifications of residues by chemical or enzymatic means.

These changes represent, in fact, fundamental physiological processes necessary in order for the organism to function normally; however, by the generation of neo-epitopes, these changes can determine the formation of anti-modified protein antibodies (AMPA), for example ACPA, in subjects that are genetically susceptible and are subjected to certain risk factors [10].

As a chronic inflammatory disease, some of the characteristics and pathogenic processes of RA mirror those of periodontitis, both of which eventually result in the progressive destruction of bone. The profound interdependence between these two diseases is the result of common genetic and environmental risk factors, including HLA-DRB1 gene expression, smoking, and other exogenous risk factors such as nutrition, socioeconomic status, and psychological factors (stress). Despite the obvious differences in etiology, there is evidence linking the two diseases, clinically, epidemiologically, serologically and experimentally [11].

2. Immunomodulatory medication in rheumatoid arthritis and its effect on periodontal disease

Given the similarities between the pathogenic aspects of periodontitis and rheumatoid arthritis, it is pertinent that the therapeutic options available for rheumatoid arthritis be known in the periodontal research community but also by periodontal specialists that have rheumatoid arthritis patients in treatment. Although the early mechanisms that result in impaired immune tolerance and the progression of clinical signs and symptoms of rheumatoid arthritis are unknown, the inflammatory cascade plays a key role in all stages of rheumatoid arthritis pathogenesis, from autoimmunity to joint localization and joint destruction [12].

There are several treatment options available for patients with RA, imposed by international treatment guides that are independent of the oral and periodontal status, and these can include physical therapy, lifestyle changes such as diet and exercise in an effort to diminish joint stress, medication and even surgery. Among drugs the most common prescribed are non-steroidal anti-inflammatory drugs (NSAIDs) and so called anti-rheumatic disease-modifying drugs (DMARDs) [13].

The term DMARDs is used to name a group of drugs that are generally unrelated, but differ from NSAIDs (that have the purpose of reducing inflammation but not of treating RA) and also differ from steroids, that reduce the immune and inflammatory response but do not slow the progression of the disease. In other words, while NSAIDs and steroids are used to control RA symptoms, only DMARDS influences the progression of the disease [14].

DMARDS act as immunosuppressive and immunomodulatory agents and are divided in two major groups: conventional and biologic. Regarding the mechanism of action, each DMARD is unique and it is by consequence of the specific pathways it affects in the inflammatory cascade. In clinical practice the most frequently used conventional DMARDS are methotrexate, hydroxychloroquine, leflunomide, and sulfasalazine [13].

Biologics are the other major class of DMARDS made accessible for the first time in the early 90's and are frequently prescribed when conventional therapy is not effective, objectified by clinical or radiological disease progression and on-going disease activity. This type of medication is highly specific and it targets a particular immune system pathway. Biological DMARDs include a number of anti-cytokine agents that block the activity of specific cytokines and are usually monoclonal antibodies that bind to the target cytokine [14]. Examples of biologics include TNF inhibitors (adalimumab, infliximab, certolizumab, etanercept), anti-CD20 (rituximab), anti-CD80 and anti CD-86 (abatacept), anti-IL-6 (tocilizumab, sirukumab), anti-IL-17 (secukinumab, ixekizumab) and Janus Kinase (JAK) inhibitors (tofacitinib, baricitinib) to name a few [13].

DMARDs determine the reduction of the level of inflammatory markers such as CRP and rheumatoid factor (RF), the rate of erythrocyte sedimentation (ESR), and also cartilage and bone damage. In the treatment of rheumatoid arthritis, therapy with biological DMARDs is often prescribed in combination with a conventional agent in those patients that presented a limited response to conventional antirheumatic disease-modifying therapy.

Tumor necrosis factor-alpha (TNF-α) is a particularly important proinflammatory mediator and therefore, one of the primary objectives of the development of anti-cytokine therapies that have been introduced in the treatment of rheumatoid arthritis has been the development of anti-TNFα agents. Other cytokines that play a role in the pathogenesis of rheumatoid arthritis include interleukin-1 (IL-1), interleukin-6, interleukin-17, interleukin-15 and more recently interleukin-23 [14].

Additional studies are needed to better understand these mechanisms and help maintain general health, oral health parameters requiring close monitoring in RA patients.

Periodontal disease therapy by modulating the host response is a high interest subject in periodontology and several classes of drugs have been proposed to fulfil this desiderate, some of them are even used in the treatment of rheumatoid arthritis. Amongst the potential host modulator drugs we mention NSAIDs, corticosteroids, conventional synthetic disease modifiers (DMARDs), matrix-metalloproteinase (MMP) inhibitors, clinically modified tetracyclines, anti-cytokines and biologic therapies, lipid mediators of resolution of inflammation, small molecule compounds, histone diacetylase inhibitors, RANKL inhibitors, bisphosphonates, Toll-like receptor inhibitors and also the combined anti-inflammatory and antibacterial approach [13].

Considering the common proinflammatory pathways between the two diseases, interactions with the immune system and the additional systemic inflammatory burden that accompanies periodontal disease we wanted to assess to what degree specific rheumatoid arthritis drug therapy influences periodontal status and if there is any difference regarding treatment combinations on oral status amongst RA subjects. Furthermore, we wanted to verify whether there is any difference in the severity of rheumatic disease and disease activity according to oral health status.

To accomplish this task we conducted a study on 220 patients with a verified diagnosis of rheumatoid arthritis in which we analysed the local inflammatory status, by evaluating the Quigley Hein (QH) indices, the Lőe and Silness gingival index (GI), the papillary bleeding index (PBI), Probing Depth (PD) and the Community Periodontal Index of Treatment Needs (CPITN), accompanied by a detailed assessment of the systemic status in patients with rheumatoid arthritis, including indexes of rheumatic disease activity but also systemic non-specific inflammatory markers such as C reactive protein (CRP) and erythrocyte sedimentation rate (ESR) [15].

There is no consensus in the literature regarding the severity of periodontal disease in rheumatoid arthritis patients, however authors agree that the percentage of moderate to severe periodontitis is higher in RA patients when compared to systemically healthy controls with periodontitis.

In our study, following the periodontal examination, 149 of the total 220 patients with rheumatic pathology were diagnosed with moderate and severe periodontitis, so from a percentage point of view we can say that 67.72% of the analysed group have moderate to severe periodontal damage. These results are similar with those from Erikson [16] who found a percentage of 75% out of 45 patients had moderate or severe periodontitis, Rodríguez-Lozano [17] on the other hand, reported 45% of 187 RA subjects had severe periodontitis and finally another study reported an astounding 98% (out of 168 subjects) were suffering from moderate to severe periodontal disease [18].

Other than the oral status, from a systemic, rheumatic point of view we analysed the following disease markers:

2.1 Clinical status of rheumatic disease (Stage I to IV)

Stage 1: It is the incipient stage and involves the initial joint capsule inflammation and synovial tissue swelling; causes evident symptoms of joint oedema, stiffness and pain.

Stage 2: Cartilage deterioration due to synovium inflammation which causes more important limitation of mobility.

Stage 3: Due to the substantial inflammation of the synovial tissue the bone is affected, not only the cartilaginous tissue. Subjectively, pain increases marked oedema, loss of muscle vigour and mobility, furthermore, deformations of the joint may appear.

Stage 4: In the ultimate stage of rheumatic disease the joints are no longer functional and the inflammation stops. Subjects experience loss of mobility, stifness, oedema and pain.

On the studied cases, among the patients with rheumatoid arthritis, the distribution of the subjects on the four stages was: stage I - 0.9%, stage II - 11.8%, stage III - 50.9% and stage IV - 36.4%.

2.2 VAS score (Visual Analogue Scale) for pain assessment

VAS (analogue visual scale) is a measuring instrument, often used in epidemiological and clinical research to measure the intensity or frequency of various symptoms. Using a ruler, the score is determined by measuring the distance (mm) on the 10 cm line between the "pain-free" point and extreme pain, providing a range of scores between 0-100.

The VAS pain assessment score ranged from 10-90, with a mean value of 36.55 ± 21.17, which included the study group with a moderate perception of pain.

2.3 DAS28

The DAS28 score (disease activity score) is a measure of disease activity in rheumatoid arthritis, 28 representing the examined joints. The range of measures of disease activity in RA is wide and it includes: assesement of joints for oedema and tumefaction, overall pain scores and general condition, inflammation serum biomarkers (eg ESR - erythrocyte sedimentation rate and CRP - C reactive protein), questionnaires, radiographic examinations, nuclear magnetic resonance and ultrasound.

DAS28 is a composite score, the results are entered into a complex mathematical formula to produce the overall score of disease activity. A DAS28 greater than 5.1 involves active disease, less than 3.2 decreased disease activity, and less than 2.6 remission.

2.4 Rheumatoid factor (RF)

For 86.4% of patients, rheumatoid factor was found to be positive. The correlation of rheumatoid factor positivity with the staging of rheumatoid arthritis showed that 52.6% of patients with positive rheumatoid factor were in stage III of the disease, and 36.8% in stage IV ($p = 0.014$).

2.5 AntiCCP antibodies (ACPA)

63.6% of patients had antiCCP antibodies. The correlation of the presence of antiCCP Ac with the staging of rheumatoid arthritis showed that 51.4% of patients with positive antiCCP Ac were in stage III of the disease, and 34.3% in stage IV ($p = 0.451$).

Among the associated comorbidities, on the studied cases, most frequently, the presence of hypertension (54.5%) and osteoporosis (31.8%) was noticed.

Regarding medication for RA, we observed that the most frequently prescribed were mainly the following: Leflunomide (46.4%) and Rituximab (44.5%), and Methotrexate 23.6%, of all cases, followed by 18.2% Adalimumab and 15.5% Tocilizumab. However, it is important to specify that the majority of patients have a combined medication of 2 drugs. The most frequent combination for our group are the following synthetic DMARDS combined with biological DMARDS: Methotrexate + Rituximab (11.8%) and Methotrexate + Adalimumab (6.4%) respectively. Another popular scheme was Leflunomide + Rituximab (20.9%), Leflunomide + Adalimumab (18.2%) and Leflunomide + Etanercept (11.8%).

When we analysed the correlation between ESR and medication, we observed that the lowest mean level is found in patients treated with Hydroxychloroquine + Rituximab and Methotrexate + Adalimumab, and the highest was recorded in subjects who received Hydroxychloroquine + Tocilizumab.

Regarding the classic inflammatory marker (CRP), the lowest mean level was recorded in patients treated with Methotrexate + Adalimumab, and the highest in subjects treated with Hydroxychloroquine + Tocilizumab.

Measurement of periodontal indexes revealed the lowest mean Quigley Hein index was in subjects under a combination of Sulfasalazine and Rituximab therapy, and the highest scores were for Leflunomid and Etanercept combination.

GI index mean was lowest in subjects under Methotrexate or Leflunomide and Adalimumab combination, on the other hand, the highest was observed in the Leflunomide or Methotrexate and Rituximab combination. The lowest mean level of PBI is observed in patients treated with Leflunomid + Etanercept, and the highest in patients treated with Leflunomid + Rituximab. Regarding another specific clinical periodontal marker, the mean CPITN level did not differ significantly depending on the combined synthetic and biological DMARDS treatment.

In our study, RF was registered in a positive proportion of 86.4%, and the correlation of rheumatoid factor positivity with the staging of rheumatoid arthritis showed that as the joint damage is in a more advanced stage, so does the probability of the presence of RF.

In a systematic review in 2016, Fuggle et al. revealed that there is an increased risk of bleeding on probing (BOP) in patients with RA compared to subjects without joint damage ($p = 0.05$), and in terms of oral hygiene parameters, the gingival index (GI) was significantly higher in level in RA compared to healthy controls; not the same was recorded in the plaque index analysis, another parameter of oral hygiene analysed in that study [19].

In 2015, Araújo et al. published a review of studies investigating the relationship between RA and periodontitis, in which articles were selected from 2012, including eight epidemiological studies, four periodontal intervention studies and five studies that investigated the role of inflammatory mediators in both diseases, highlighting that 21 of studies confirmed the association of the two entities, by statistical analysis, while 3 studies demonstrated an association by descriptive analysis [20].

Two studies from 2013, Bıyıkoğlu et al., and Erciyas et al., respectively, analysed the effect of non-surgical periodontal therapy on the DAS 28 score, both observing a reduction of this parameter, with values that remained stable post-treatment [21, 22]. Moreover, Erciyas et al. also analysed other parameters such as ESR and CRP and noted that the changes were more prominent in the group with high disease activity compared to the group with low activity [22].

In our study, the modified values of the analysed oral and periodontal health indices were significantly correlated with stage III or IV of RA. Most likely, the motor restrictions encountered by these patients make it difficult to achieve adequate oral hygiene; the burden of the disease in general affecting the quality of life can be additional factors in the subsistence of a poor periodontal status.

The analysed data in our study show that as the rheumatic damage increases, the oral status is altered in direct proportion to all indices, but especially in terms of GI and PBI which are relevant oral indicators in case of an exacerbated systemic inflammatory status, a fact confirmed by Payne in 2015 [23]. Our study thus represents an opening to the clinical correlation between periodontal inflammatory status and the degree of rheumatic damage.

Several studies have shown that non-surgical periodontal treatment is able to reduce serum levels of TNF-α, IL-1β, IL-6, IL-10, MMP-8 and C-reactive protein and to modulate RA activity in patients with moderate to severe periodontitis [24, 25].

Modulation of T cell activation has provided another therapeutic target in RA with the use of abatacept, and inhibition of alveolar bone loss has suggested that treatment with RA may also improve the progression of periodontitis [26]; however, this is only an experimental study, without clinical data on human subjects available just yet.

In conclusion, there is no definitive data in human subjects to evaluate the effects of DMARDs on periodontitis due to the small number of patients studied and the lack of randomized, double-blind, placebo-controlled studies. The use of anti-TNF antibodies did not consistently prevent alveolar bone loss and generated aggravated or improved gingival inflammation, depending on the specific drug used. It is not clear whether these divergent results reflect differences in the structure of the studied anti-TNF studies. To date, the most impressive beneficial effect has been observed in inhibiting IL-6 related to tocilizumab, an IL-6 receptor antibody. Subsequent studies with tocilizumab, as well as observations with anti-IL-6 antibodies, may elucidate the importance of this cytokine in the pathogenesis of periodontitis.

The biological rationale for using DMARDS as a modulator of periodontitis expression in animals was confirmed by studies showing that mice deficient in the TN55-α p55 receptor developed less severe periodontal inflammation (reduced bone loss and a low inflammatory response) in response to inoculation with *A. actinomycetemcomitans* [27]. Using the same model of experimental periodontitis induced by *A. actinomycetemcomitans*, researchers found that antigen-induced arthritis exacerbated alveolar bone loss, while anti-TNF-α therapies improved the development of periodontitis [28].

To date, most research on the use of anti-cytokine therapies for periodontitis in humans has been limited to small clinical trials evaluating periodontal status in patients with rheumatoid arthritis under treatment. The findings from these studies tended to be inconsistent and somewhat confusing, probably due to the small number of patients with a variety of periodontal conditions, selected due to the primary inclusion criterion (anti-cytokine therapy for rheumatoid arthritis), different from the recruitment situation which was a targeted and deliberate one, in accordance with their periodontal status.

A study of three groups of patients (one with autoimmune diseases including RA who were not treated with anti-TNF-α therapy, the second with RA who received anti-TNF-α therapy and the healthy control group without autoimmune disease, and no anti-TNF-α treatment) identified that patients with autoimmune disease who did not receive anti-TNF-α treatment had severe levels of gingival inflammation, bleeding on probing, higher mean probing depths and higher concentrations of TNF-α in the crevicular fluid compared to subjects in the other two groups [29]. This research has shown that patients with autoimmune disorders (including RA) have a much more severe periodontal inflammation than patients who do not suffer from autoimmune diseases, anti-TNF-α therapy reducing inflammation in periodontal tissues.

In our study, the combination of methotrexate and adalimumab had the lowest ESR and CRP values, consistent with multiple studies attesting to the systemic anti-inflammatory effect of methotrexate in particular [30, 31]. The combinations of leflunomide and adalimumab, as well as leflunomide with etanercept, recorded the most marked decrease in both rheumatic disease and oral health indices, results similar to those of McInnes and Schett in 2017 which identified that patients with rheumatoid arthritis who received anti-TNF-α treatment showed statistically significant improvements in probe depth, probe bleeding, and gingival inflammation compared to patients who did not receive anti-TNF-α therapy after non-surgical periodontal treatment [32].

The combination of leflunomide with rituximab or methotrexate with rituximab was associated in our study with the highest values of GI and PBI indices, data that coincides with similar studies in the literature [33]. Most likely these values are increased due to the inhibitory action of rituximab on CD20 B lymphocytes. When this drug binds to CD20 it triggers cellular death, which in time leads to almost complete depletion of peripheral B cells. Long-lived plasma cells that do not express this protein (CD20) are not directly affected by rituximab treatment, since this therapeutic agent only targets CD20 expressing cells.

Through our studies in which we analyzed the potential relation between the medication administered in rheumatoid arthritis and oral health indexes we could not confirm an effect on oral status of patients treated with conventional and synthetic DMARDS combination. An interesting finding is that patients treated with biologics had lower oral health indexes, thus a lower inflammation of the periodontal tissues. We could observe the beneficial effect of TNF-α inhibitors which although administered systemically have a local effect [15].

Adequate oral health measures should be part of the routine recommendations offered to RA patients. Adequate periodontal diagnosis by a periodontal specialist is necessary to determine the optimum course of treatment. Reducing the oral inflammatory contribution to the total inflammatory load as a result of the favourable outcome of periodontal treatment is an important desideratum. Maintaining the complete health of patients with RA must be a collaborative effort. This partnership dentist - rheumatologist will certainly influence the oral and overall health of these patients.

There is a strong association between RA and periodontitis. Interventions to prevent, reduce or treat periodontitis in arthritis patients will certainly promote better health status for these patients.

3. Periodontopathogenic bacteria in rheumatoid arthritis patients

Several studies have shown that periodontitis is more common in patients with active RA compared to healthy people; also, the prevalence of RA is higher in people with periodontitis compared to subjects without periodontitis [34]. In addition, the course of periodontal disease in patients with RA was more severe, regardless of age, sex, ethnicity, or smoking history [5].

Despite all the evidence supporting an association between these two diseases, the pathophysiological mechanisms have not yet been fully defined. In order to elucidate the clinical, biochemical and immunological interrelationship, it is necessary to perform longitudinal, prospective, large multi-center clinical trials to eliminate the risk of bias given by medication or associated pathology, oral hygiene, socioeconomic status, sex, age and vicious habits such as smoking.

Regarding the hypothesis of a causal link between periodontal disease and rheumatoid arthritis, where periodontitis is the determining factor, there are several theories in place.

The first one would be the release of extracellular traps by neutrophils (NET), in response to infection with *P. gingivalis*, structures characterized by active proteases and PAD. The concomitant action of these enzymes generates citrullinate epitopes and triggers the synthesis of ACPA. The production of citrullinate epitopes is accelerated by the synergistic action of gingipain and peptidilarginine deiminase of *P. gingivalis* (PPAD). Certain proteins from bacteria have the ability to mimic human proteins (bacteria enolase is similar to α-enolase in humans) on a molecular level and is thought to participate in the loss of immune tolerance to the organisms own molecules. Citrullinated epitopes in articular joints are the target of a secondary signal which causes increased generation of ACPA and rheumatoid factor, thus inducing immune complexes accumulation.

A second pathway would be neutrophil necrosis in the periodontal pocket, thus releasing danger-associated molecular patterns (DAMP) which circulate in the blood stream and exacerbate inflammation, both locally and systemically.

The third pathway is mediated by virulence factors expressed by *P. gingivalis*, such as lipopolysaccharides, fimbriae, gingipains, and lipoproteins, which are recognized by Toll-like receptors, protease-activated receptors, and/or NOD2 receptors on gingival and phagocytic epithelial cells. In response to pathogens, host cells release cytokines and chemokines that activate the complement system, RANKL, and promote T-helper cell differentiation, thus contributing to osteoclastogenesis [11].

PPAD-dependent disorder of immune tolerance caused by *P. gingivalis* can be considered the causal link between periodontal infection and RA. However, endogenous PADs are also important because they have very high values in chronic infections, such as periodontitis [35].

Recent findings make it clear that these two pathologies are intimately connected not only by similarities in pathogenic mechanisms and genetic and environmental risk factors, but also by data provided by cohort studies showing that periodontitis precedes the development of RA and that periodontal disease in individuals who develop RA at a later date correlates positively with ACPA levels; all of these are important arguments that support a causal interrelationship.

In this disease model, the inflamed periodontal tissue is the site where immune tolerance to citrulline epitopes is surpassed and ACPA production begins, this theory being verified in animal studies and is consistent with the paradigm according to which ACPAs are generated in mucosal surfaces, their formation preceding the clinical symptoms of rheumatic pathology for many years. In this case, periodontal pathogens can be considered direct determinants of autoimmune reactions, this being supported by case-control studies showing the generation of ACPAs and other mucosal surfaces such as the lungs and gastrointestinal tract, illustrating a heterogeneous picture of bacterial-host interactions within the human microbiome complexity.

In order to clarify this issue we conducted a study [36] on 19 patients with rheumatoid arthritis in order to identify bacterial DNA, by PCR analysis, in the subgingival dental plaque and serum in patients affected by rheumatoid arthritis and periodontitis. The patients were diagnosed with refractory severe rheumatoid arthritis, in spite of intensive DMARDs treatment which included methotrexate, sulfasalazine, leflunomide and chloroquine. Patients who had other comorbidities were excluded from the study, as well as pregnant or nursing women, antibiotic therapy or periodontal treatment in the last 3 months prior to the study.

All patients were treated with DMARDs most of them also benefited from NSAID medication and low-dose steroids. The diagnosis of periodontitis was determined by measuring the depth of the periodontal pocket (PD) and the clinical loss of attachment (CAL).

The disease time course of rheumatoid arthritis was 8.71 (± 5.99) years, with a range of 0.5-20 years from the initial clinical diagnosis of rheumatoid arthritis. Chronic periodontitis was the most common type detected, whereas the aggressive form was present in only 5% of analyzed subjects, although the sample size for this study was small.

When we investigated the stage of periodontal disease, the most commonly represented for our study group was the severe stage (42.2%), whereas moderate (36.8%) and mild (21.1%) were present to a lesser degree. These percentages are similar to other studies [17]. The average overall depth of the pocket was 3.9 mm, however, taking into account the biggest depth of the pocket of each dental unit, the average was 4.2 mm. In terms of loss of attachment, the upper molars were the most affected (3.85 mm average).

The periodontopathogenic load was considerable for this group of patients, as nearly 100% of the subgingival samples were positive for bacteria and the venous blood samples in 84.2%. In subgingival samples *P. Intermedia* (100%), *T. denticola* (84.2%) and *P. gingivalis* (78.9%) were the most frequently observed, and in venous blood *P. Intermedia* 73.6% and *P. gingivalis* 42.1%.

The least common species detected was *A. actinomycetemcomitans* (15.7%). When we compare the two types of samples we can observe no significant statistical differences regarding *A. actinomycetemcomitans* and *P. gingivalis* between the samples, other hand, other analyzed species did show statistically significant differences.

In this study, only 19 patients were included due to the difficulty of finding patients who met the inclusion criteria. Patients with refractory rheumatoid arthritis treated with DMARDs were selected because this condition was necessary to obtain a serum sample with significant detectable characteristics. Most patients were female (84.2%), and was consistent with the information that rheumatoid arthritis affects women more than men [4].

It is justified to argue that the lower concentration of bacteria DNA in the venous blood is due to the renal filtration. Other authors found similar data by using a checkerboard DNA-DNA-hybridization set up and bacterial DNA was detected in 100% of analyzed serum samples thus implicating a continual aggression of oral pathogenic bacteria in joint disease [37].

In our study the most frequent bacterial species identified in venous blood were *P. gingivalis, T. denticola and P. intermedia,* the first two belonging to the red complex, and more often than not, correlated with a highly distructive periodontal disease pattern. On the other hand, *A. actinomycetemcomitans* which is thought to be mainly responsible for a more rapidly progressive type periodontitis, was less frequently detected. The reason could be that only one patient was affected. These data are consistent with previous reports.

The fact that *A. actinomycetemcomitans* and *P. gingivalis* did not show statistically significant differences between samples suggests that this could be a significant bacterial association for rheumatoid arthritis patients because the same bacteria species detected in serum were present also in bacterial plaque samples. On the other hand, there were statistical differences between samples for *P. intermedia*, *T. forsythia*, *P. nigrescens* and *T. denticola*, suggesting a more minor role for these periodontal pathogens.

The tooth associated microflora has been extensively studied. The presence of *Porphyromonas gingivalis, Tannerella forsythia, Aggregatibacter actinomycetemcomitans* in the gingival sulcus poses an increased risk for developement and severity of periodontitis. Healthy versus diseased periodontal sites are different in terms of microbiological composition. The healthy sulcus has a lower bacterial load and also less morphological types, whereas the periodontal pocket is a complex microenvironment with an abundance of microorganisms that are mostly anaerobic gram-negative periodontopathogens [38].

Another interesting result of our study is the fact that all bacterial serum positive patients were also positive for the same bacteria in the subgingival plaque, thus proving a direct link to the oral cavity. On a similar note, some studies in the literature discovered antibodies against *P. intermedia* in periodontal tissues and in the synovium of subjects with rheumatoid arthritis. Moreover, the induction of proinflammatory cytokines in the synovial tissue of rheumatoid arthritis subjects is exacerbated by elevated heat shock protein 70 expressions precipitated by specific stress stimulating factors [39]. This confirms our results which place *P. intermedia* as the most frequently identified bacteria in rheumatoid arthritis subjects.

Whole-genome shotgun (WGS) sequencing is a newer technique that analyzes bacteria genomes with important roles in a metagenomic sample. Through this method a more global, complex image of the microbial ecosystem is obtained because it examines the metabolic pathways and the complete set of genes pertaining to the community.

A recent study determined that species of *Prevotella* (microorganisms of oral origin) are increased in the gut microbiome of rheumatoid arthritis subjects [40]. These results are sustained by another study performed on patients in preclinical rheumatoid arthritis stages that reported high numbers of *Prevotella spp* in these patients [41]. Thus colonization by oral microorganisms of the gut could be linked to the pathogenesis of rheumatic diseases.

Metagenomic studies are an important research direction that could establish other links in the periodontitis-rheumatoid arthritis binome, and have the potential to better determine the microbial diversity and ecology in these subjects.

Considering the presented data it is fair to articulate an important role of oral pathogens DNA in the pathogenesis of rheumatic diseases. The migration of DNA from periodontal pockets to the joints could be by means of the free bacterial DNA. This information can be valuable for future studies to elucidate whether periodontal pathogenic DNA might be a possible trigger for rheumatoid arthritis development.

4. Future research possibilities in the rheumatoid arthritis-periodontitis interface

Host response modulation therapy is a highly researched topic in the scientific literature, and more specifically, when referring to the management of periodontal disease, a number of potential drugs have been considered for treatment. The first studies on this topic date back 30 years ago and they analyzed the intake of nonsteroidal anti-inflammatory drugs for the minimization of alveolar bone loss. Due to the fact that they were prescribed for long periods of time, important undesirable side effects were associated with their administration, and thus precluding their use as adjunctive therapy for periodontitis; in other words, the associated risks far outweigh any potential benefits in reducing alveolar bone resorption.

In the 1990s, a new wave of research investigated the use of tetracycline compounds, specifically doxycycline, after identifying its efficacy as an inhibitor of matrix metalloproteinases. Randomized controlled clinical trials have confirmed a benefit of using subantimicrobial doses (20 mg twice daily for 3 months) as an adjunct to conventional non-surgical treatment, with no evidence of undesirable side effects. To date, this dose of doxycycline is the only drug therapy widely available, authorized as a host modulating agent for use in the treatment of periodontal disease. However, not all studies have shown the same clear benefit as seen in large-scale clinical trials, and there are still uncertainties about the category of patients for whom such treatment would provide feasible results, and can be anticipated in routine periodontal practice [42].

Anti-cytokine therapies have a proven efficacy in the management of rheumatoid arthritis and, given the similarities between the pathogenesis of rheumatoid arthritis and periodontitis, researchers' interest in anti-cytokine therapies as potential modulators of the host response in the treatment of periodontitis is justified. However, there are concerns associated with their use due to well-documented side effects, such as an increased risk of infection and malignancy [43]. In addition, cytokines function in complex cellular and molecular networks that integrate aspects of innate and adaptive immunity that are still challenging to assess in their complexity.

Similar to other autoimmune and chronic inflammatory conditions, our knowledge of all cytokine functions in periodontitis is far from exhaustive, and simple inhibition of a certain cytokine may not determine a clinically significant impact on the researched pathological condition. This is due to the fact that a great deal of cytokines and biomolecules exert a similar effect on the cells they interact with, thus it is possible that inhibition of a certain cytokine could have little to no detectable influence on a pathological condition. This is by consequence of other cytokines which have a similar function to the one that was repressed. In addition, even though animal models may suggest certain anti-cytokine drugs that could ameliorate, or even amend, the course of a disease such as rheumatoid arthritis, they cannot predict exactly whether the same efficacy can be obtained in human or individual patient studies.

In the treatment of rheumatoid arthritis, inhibition of TNF-α with antagonist therapies plus methotrexate has clearly demonstrated clinical improvements, due to the fact that this molecule is of major importance in the pathogenesis of the disease. Moreover, anti-TNF-α therapy in patients with rheumatoid arthritis results in a reduction of other pro-inflammatory mediators, such as IL-1β and IL-6, leading to an improvement of the anti-inflammatory effect [32]. Even so, the use of these therapies does not lead to complete eradication of the disease, and success factors are assessed using composite scales that take into account not only the improvement quantified in percentage in the clinical signs and symptoms of the disease, but also the high cost and high risk of significant side effects.

The method of administration (typically repeated subcutaneous injections or intravenous infusions) is another limiting factor; however, it is possible that future generations of anti-TNF-α agents (possibly even locally released) may have a much higher impact on the treatment of periodontitis.

Compounds with small molecules, for example histone deacetylase inhibitors, could potentially successfully manage certain pathological conditions that determine bone resorption. Considering the fact that they have an inhibitory effect on the activity of osteoclasts they could be coupled with anti-inflammatory drugs for the minimization of inflammation and osseous resorption. Another area of interest is the advancement of synthetically produced specific deacetylase inhibitors targeting the histone diacetylases that are implicated in the dysfunction process [44].

On the other hand, the potential side-effects on other cellular processes are not to be ignored and supplementary studies characterizing the risk-benefit ratio are paramount. Another potentially confounding or even aggravating factor may be the difference in mechanism of action of biological therapies in animal versus human subjects which could have unfortunate consequences when applied for the first time. In spite of all this, these compounds are currently being evaluated in early-stage clinical trials as a treatment plan in neoplasms and show promising preliminary results in terms of effectiveness and toleration [45].

A newly emerging class of drugs that shows great promise in the adjunctive treatment of periodontal disease is pro-resolution lipid mediators. A major benefit of these endogenous compounds is that they are generated as a physiological response to inflammation (resolution agonists), contrary to inhibitors of inflammation that may imperil host defense [46]. The development of drugs that mimic the actions of endogenous mediators that lead to the resolution of inflammation could be useful in the treatment of a number of chronic inflammatory diseases, including periodontitis; obviously, efforts to demonstrate their safety and effectiveness will be commensurate.

Therefore, the immunomodulatory properties of a number of molecules and classes of drugs are being investigated, with the precise purpose of evaluating the applicability in the treatment of periodontal disease. The challenge at hand that still remains is to capitalize on the information gained from fundamental studies and animal model experiments in order to promote the development and evaluation of these compounds as novel therapeutic options. Furthermore, assessment of the risk/benefit ratio driven by large scale clinical use, taking into account the potential diversity in the response profile in-between subjects, interactions with other medication and potential adverse effects is imperative. Nonetheless, it is highly possible that in the future a new series of modular anti-inflammatory and pro-resolving therapies will be identified; these therapeutic agents could have direct relevance as adjuvants in the treatment of periodontal disease.

5. Conclusions

Significant evidence suggests that citrullination may bind periodontal disease to rheumatoid arthritis. Genetic factors drive host responses to chronic diseases with complex pathogenesis. In the future, more effective therapeutic approaches will include multiple synergistic therapies to modulate the host response, combined with treatments that target microbial etiology. Further studies are needed to better understand these mechanisms and help maintain overall health, with oral health parameters requiring close monitoring in patients with RA.

Given the similarities between aspects of the pathogenesis of periodontitis and rheumatoid arthritis, it is relevant that in the periodontology research community there is a great deal of interest for optimizing the treatment options applicable in rheumatoid arthritis patients. Even though impaired immune tolerance and introduction of symptoms in rheumatoid arthritis have yet to be fully comprehended, it is evident that concerning the pathogenesis of this disease the inflammatory cascade is the leading actor from start to finish; beginning with the initiation of autoimmunity, to the subsequent synovial localization, and culminating in the joint and bone tissue destruction.

Interventions to improve oral pathology can have direct and indirect systemic benefits. Considerations which must be taken into account include the patient's ability to maintain adequate oral hygiene, xerostomia and associated complications due to drug intake or disease course, the patient's susceptibility to infections, alterations in hemostasis, and drug mechanism of action and interactions.

Conflict of interest

The authors declare no conflict of interest.

Author details

Maria-Alexandra Martu[1*], Elena Rezus[1], Diana Tatarciuc[1], Ionut Luchian[1], Irina-Georgeta Sufaru[1], George-Alexandru Maftei[1], Dorin Gheorghe[2], Liliana Pasarin[1], Sorina Mihaela Solomon[1] and Liliana Georgeta Foia[1]

1 University of Medicine and Pharmacy "Grigore T. Popa", Iasi, Romania

2 University of Medicine and Pharmacy Craiova, Romania

*Address all correspondence to: alexandra_martu@yahoo.com

References

[1] Monsarrat P, Blaizot A, Kemoun P, Ravaud P, Nabet C, Sixou M, et al. Clinical research activity in periodontalmedicine: a systematic mapping of trial registers. J Clin Periodontol. 2016;43(5):390-400. doi:10.1111/jcpe.12534.

[2] Loos BG. Periodontal medicine: work in progress! J Clin Periodontol. 2016;43(6):470-1. doi:10.1111/jcpe.12550

[3] Zenobia C, Hajishengallis G. Basic biology and role of interleukin-17 in immunity and inflammation. Periodontology 2000. 2015 Oct 1;69(1):142-59.

[4] Catrina AI, Svensson CI, Malmström V, Schett G, Klareskog L. Mechanisms leading from systemic autoimmunity to joint-specific disease in rheumatoid arthritis. Nature Reviews Rheumatology. 2017 Feb;13(2):79.

[5] Mikuls TR, Payne JB, Deane KD, Thiele GM. Autoimmunity of the lung and oral mucosa in a multisystem inflammatory disease: The spark that lights the fire in rheumatoid arthritis?. Journal of Allergy and Clinical Immunology. 2016 Jan 1;137(1):28-34.

[6] Rosenbaum JT, Asquith MJ. The microbiome: a revolution in treatment for rheumatic diseases?. Current rheumatology reports. 2016 Oct 1;18(10):62.

[7] Montgomery AB, Kopec J, Shrestha L, Thezenas ML, Burgess-Brown NA, Fischer R, Yue WW, Venables PJ. Crystal structure of Porphyromonas gingivalis peptidylarginine deiminase: implications for autoimmunity in rheumatoid arthritis. Annals of the Rheumatic Diseases. 2016 Jun 1;75(6):1255-61

[8] Gawron K, Montgomery A, Łazarz-Bartyzel K, Bereta G, Chomyszyn-Gajewska M, Venables P, Potempa J. Porphyromonas gingivalis peptidyl arginine deiminase: A Unique bacterial PAD with implications for periodontal disease and rheumatoid Arthritis. InProtein Deimination in Human Health and Disease 2017 (pp. 99-135). Springer, Cham.

[9] Muller S, Radic M. Citrullinated autoantigens: from diagnostic markers to pathogenetic mechanisms. Clinical reviews in allergy & immunology. 2015 Oct 1;49(2):232-9.

[10] Trouw LA, Rispens T, Toes RE. Beyond citrullination: other post-translational protein modifications in rheumatoid arthritis. Nature Reviews Rheumatology. 2017 Jun;13(6):331.

[11] Potempa J, Mydel P, Koziel J. The case for periodontitis in the pathogenesis of rheumatoid arthritis. Nature Reviews Rheumatology. 2017 Oct;13(10):606.

[12] Schmickler J, Rupprecht A, Patschan S, Patschan D, Müller GA, Haak R, Mausberg RF, Schmalz G, Kottmann T, Ziebolz D. Cross-Sectional Evaluation of Periodontal Status and Microbiologic and Rheumatoid Parameters in a Large Cohort of Patients With Rheumatoid Arthritis. Journal of periodontology. 2017 Apr;88(4):368-79.

[13] Conigliaro P, Triggianese P, De Martino E, Fonti GL, Chimenti MS, Sunzini F, Viola A, Canofari C, Perricone R. Challenges in the treatment of rheumatoid arthritis. Autoimmunity reviews. 2019 Jul 1;18(7):706-13.

[14] Kerschbaumer, A., Sepriano, A., Smolen, J.S., van der Heijde, D., Dougados, M., van Vollenhoven, R., McInnes, I.B., Bijlsma, J.W., Burmester, G.R., de Wit, M. and Falzon, L., 2020. Efficacy of pharmacological treatment in rheumatoid arthritis: a systematic literature research informing the 2019

update of the EULAR recommendations for management of rheumatoid arthritis. Annals of the Rheumatic Diseases, 79(6), pp.744-759.

[15] Martu MA, Rezus E, Popa C, Solomon SM, Luchian I, Pendefunda AC, Sioustis I, Anton D, Martu S, Foia L. Correlations between systemic therapy with conventional (synthetic) and biological DMARDS, rheumatoid arthritis and periodontal indices of chronic periodontitis. Romanian Journal of Oral Rehabilitation. 2018 Oct 1;10(4).

[16] Eriksson K, Fei G, Lundmark A, Benchimol D, Lee L, Hu YO, Kats A, Saevarsdottir S, Catrina AI, Klinge B, Andersson AF. Periodontal health and oral microbiota in patients with rheumatoid arthritis. Journal of clinical medicine. 2019 May;8(5):630.

[17] Rodríguez-Lozano B, González-Febles J, Garnier-Rodríguez JL, Dadlani S, Bustabad-Reyes S, Sanz M, Sánchez-Alonso F, Sánchez-Piedra C, González-Dávila E, Díaz-González F. Association between severity of periodontitis and clinical activity in rheumatoid arthritis patients: a case–control study. Arthritis research & therapy. 2019 Dec;21(1):1-2.

[18] Schmickler J, Rupprecht A, Patschan S, Patschan D, Müller GA, Haak R, Mausberg RF, Schmalz G, Kottmann T, Ziebolz D. Cross-sectional evaluation of periodontal status and microbiologic and rheumatoid parameters in a large cohort of patients with rheumatoid arthritis. Journal of periodontology. 2017 Apr;88(4):368-79.

[19] Fuggle NR, Smith TO, Kaul A, Sofat N. Hand to mouth: a systematic review and meta-analysis of the association between rheumatoid arthritis and periodontitis. Frontiers in immunology. 2016 Mar 2;7:80.

[20] Araújo VM, Melo IM, Lima V. Relationship between periodontitis and rheumatoid arthritis: review of the literature. Mediators of inflammation. 2015;2015.

[21] Bıyıkoğlu B, Buduneli N, Aksu K, Nalbantsoy A, Lappin DF, Evrenosoğlu E, Kinane DF. Periodontal therapy in chronic periodontitis lowers gingival crevicular fluid interleukin-1beta and DAS28 in rheumatoid arthritis patients. Rheumatology international. 2013 Oct 1;33(10):2607-16.

[22] Erciyas K, Sezer U, Üstün K, Pehlivan Y, Kısacık B, Şenyurt SZ, Tarakçıoğlu M, Onat AM. Effects of periodontal therapy on disease activity and systemic inflammation in rheumatoid arthritis patients. Oral diseases. 2013 May;19(4):394-400.

[23] Payne JB, Golub LM, Thiele GM, Mikuls TR. The link between periodontitis and rheumatoid arthritis: a periodontist's perspective. Current oral health reports. 2015 Mar 1;2(1):20-9.

[24] Kirchner A, Jäger J, Krohn-Grimberghe B, Patschan S, Kottmann T, Schmalz G, Mausberg RF, Haak R, Ziebolz D. Active matrix metalloproteinase-8 and periodontal bacteria depending on periodontal status in patients with rheumatoid arthritis. Journal of periodontal research. 2017 Aug;52(4):745-54.

[25] Cosgarea R, Tristiu R, Dumitru RB, Arweiler NB, Rednic S, Sirbu CI, Lascu L, Sculean A, Eick S. Effects of non-surgical periodontal therapy on periodontal laboratory and clinical data as well as on disease activity in patients with rheumatoid arthritis. Clinical oral investigations. 2018 Mar 27:1-1.

[26] Weitzmann MN, Ofotokun I. Physiological and pathophysiological bone turnover—role of the immune system. Nature Reviews Endocrinology. 2016 Sep;12(9):518.

[27] Garlet GP, Cardoso CR, Campanelli AP, Ferreira BR,

Avila-Campos MJ, Cunha FQ, Silva JS. The dual role of p55 tumour necrosis factor-α receptor in Actinobacillus actinomycetemcomitans-induced experimental periodontitis: host protection and tissue destruction. Clinical & Experimental Immunology. 2007 Jan;147(1):128-38.

[28] Corrêa MG, Sacchetti SB, Ribeiro FV, Pimentel SP, Casarin RC, Cirano FR, Casati MZ. Periodontitis increases rheumatic factor serum levels and citrullinated proteins in gingival tissues and alter cytokine balance in arthritic rats. PloS one. 2017 Mar 30;12(3):e0174442.

[29] Mayer Y, Elimelech R, Balbir-Gurman A, Braun-Moscovici Y, Machtei EE. Periodontal condition of patients with autoimmune diseases and the effect of anti-tumor necrosis factor-α therapy. Journal of periodontology. 2013 Feb;84(2):136-42.

[30] Ramiro S, Sepriano A, Chatzidionysiou K, Nam JL, Smolen JS, van der Heijde D, Dougados M, van Vollenhoven R, Bijlsma JW, Burmester GR, Scholte-Voshaar M. Safety of synthetic and biological DMARDs: a systematic literature review informing the 2016 update of the EULAR recommendations for management of rheumatoid arthritis. Annals of the rheumatic diseases. 2017 Jun 1;76(6):1101-36.

[31] Orr CK, Najm A, Young F, McGarry T, Biniecka M, Fearon U, Veale DJ. The Utility and Limitations of CRP, ESR and DAS28-CRP in Appraising Disease Activity in Rheumatoid Arthritis. Frontiers in medicine. 2018;5.

[32] McInnes IB, Schett G. Pathogenetic insights from the treatment of rheumatoid arthritis. The Lancet. 2017 Jun 10;389(10086):2328-37.

[33] Ziebolz D, Rupprecht A, Schmickler J, Bothmann L, Krämer J, Patschan D, Müller GA, Mausberg RF, Schmidt J, Schmalz G, Patschan S. Association of different immunosuppressive medications with periodontal condition in patients with rheumatoid arthritis–results from a cross-sectional study. Journal of periodontology. 2018 May 22.

[34] Eriksson K, Nise L, Kats A, Luttropp E, Catrina AI, Askling J, Jansson L, Alfredsson L, Klareskog L, Lundberg K, Yucel-Lindberg T. Prevalence of periodontitis in patients with established rheumatoid arthritis: a Swedish population based case-control study. PLoS One. 2016 May 20;11(5): e0155956.

[35] Shimada A, Kobayashi T, Ito S, Okada M, Murasawa A, Nakazono K, Yoshie H. Expression of anti-Porphyromonas gingivalis peptidylarginine deiminase immunoglobulin G and peptidylarginine deiminase-4 in patients with rheumatoid arthritis and periodontitis. Journal of periodontal research. 2016 Feb 1;51(1):103-11.

[36] Martu MA, Solomon SM, Sufaru IG, Jelihovschi I, Martu S, Rezus E, Surdu AE, Onea RM, Grecu GP, Foia L. Study on the prevalence of periodontopathogenic bacteria in serum and subgingival bacterial plaque in patients with rheumatoid arthritis. Rev Chim. (Bucharest). 2017 Aug 1;68(8):1946-9.

[37] Moen K, Brun JG, Valen M, Skartveit L, Eribe EK, Olsen I, Jonsson R. Synovial inflammation in active rheumatoid arthritis and psoriatic arthritis facilitates trapping of a variety of oral bacterial DNAs. Clin Exp Rheumatol. 2006 Dec;24(6):656-3.

[38] Curtis MA, Diaz PI, Van Dyke TE. The role of the microbiota in periodontal disease. Periodontology 2000. 2020 Jun;83(1):14-25.

[39] Schenkein HA, Papapanou PN, Genco R, Sanz M. Mechanisms underlying the association between

periodontitis and atherosclerotic disease. Periodontology 2000. 2020 Jun;83(1):90-106.

[40] Kishikawa T, Maeda Y, Nii T, Motooka D, Matsumoto Y, Matsushita M, Matsuoka H, Yoshimura M, Kawada S, Teshigawara S, Oguro E. Metagenome-wide association study of gut microbiome revealed novel aetiology of rheumatoid arthritis in the Japanese population. Annals of the rheumatic diseases. 2020 Jan 1;79(1):103-11.

[41] Wells PM, Adebayo AS, Freidin MB, Finckh A, Strowig T, Lesker TR, Alpizar-Rodriguez D, Gilbert B, Kirkham B, Cope AP, Steves CJ. A polygenic risk score for rheumatoid arthritis sheds light on the Prevotella association. MedRxiv. 2019 Jan 1.

[42] Kinane DF, Stathopoulou PG, Papapanou PN. Periodontal diseases. Nature Reviews Disease Primers. 2017 Jun 22;3:17038

[43] Meyle J, Dommisch H, Groeger S, Giacaman RA, Costalonga M, Herzberg M. The innate host response in caries and periodontitis. Journal of clinical periodontology. 2017 Dec;44(12):1215-25.

[44] Grabiec AM, Potempa J. Epigenetic regulation in bacterial infections: targeting histone deacetylases. Critical reviews in microbiology. 2018 May 4;44(3):336-50.

[45] Cappelli LC, Shah AA. The relationships between cancer and autoimmune rheumatic diseases. Best Practice & Research Clinical Rheumatology. 2020 Feb 3:101472.

[46] Van Dyke TE, Sima C. Understanding resolution of inflammation in periodontal diseases: Is chronic inflammatory periodontitis a failure to resolve?. Periodontology 2000. 2020 Feb;82(1):205-13.

Chapter 8

Innate Immune Response as a New Challenge in Periodontal Inflammation

Ana Marina Andrei, Elena Cristina Andrei, Elena Camelia Stănciulescu, Mihaela Cezarina Mehedinți, Mihaela Jana Țuculină, Ileana Monica Baniță, Sandra Alice Buteică and Cătălina Gabriela Pisoschi

Abstract

Gingivitis and periodontitis are induced by numerous pathogenic microbiota hosted in the subgingival biofilm that first trigger the innate immune response. Innate immune response is part of a homeostatic system which is the first line defence and defines the host inherited resistance to infection. Both genetic and environmental factors are involved in variable individual susceptibility to inflammation of periodontal tissues. That is why, although more than 600 bacterial species have been detected in the periodontal plaque, the type of bacteria incriminated in the development of the inflammation is still unclear. Moreover, in the last decade gene polymorphisms have been largely recognised as important conditions associated with increased susceptibility to periodontal diseases. Manipulating the immune response by the development of drugs that inhibit adverse host reactions and promote beneficial effects might be of therapeutic or prophylactic importance. This work intends to assess the importance of Toll-like receptors as main effectors of the innate immune response in the triggering, maintenance and progression of periodontal inflammation, as well as of the involvement of synthetic molecules targeting TLR signalling pathways in treating periodontal diseases.

Keywords: innate immunity, toll-like receptors, periodontal inflammation, therapy

1. Introduction

The surface of the mouth is lined by the oral mucosa which was often considered to be more of a mechanic barrier than an active player involved in the modulation of the host response to various external stimuli in order to maintain mouth homeostasis.

The oral mucosa is permanently insulted by mechanic and chemical factors (like smoke, xenobiotics) as well as a plethora of microorganisms. Both the commensal and pathogen microorganisms, depending on their structure, represent triggers for the immune surveillance players hosted by the oral mucosa which have been intensively studied in the last years. Local defence in the oral cavity is provided by a complex network of cells with their receptors and molecules through which they respond to various ligands (microbial antigens, tissue degradation products, nucleic acids). The interactions between gingival resident cells and oral microbiome are characteristic of clinical gingival health and homeostasis as well as for gingival inflammation. Host defence takes place in successive, sometimes overlapping stages. The innate immune response represents a homeostatic system which is the first line defence and defines the host inherited resistance to infection.

The immune system has a hierarchical organisation, all the immune and non-immune cells involved being able to sense the pathogens through pattern recognition receptors (PRR) and then develop the immune response triggered by numerous proinflammatory mediators. PRRs detect and respond to conserved patterns originated in microorganisms and stress signals called pathogen- or damage-associated molecular patterns (PAMPS and DAMPS) [1].

Among PRRs, Toll-like receptors (TLRs) are the most intensively studied. In the oral mucosa TLRs are expressed in cells of the immune system including neutrophils, monocytes, macrophages, and not less important, dendritic cells, keratinocytes and endothelial cells [2]. TLR activation induces the local synthesis of cytokines and chemokines through different pathways. Part of these molecules are involved in the development of highly specific adaptive immunity ensured by T and B lymphocytes. Due to this ability, TLRs are considered to be the missing link between innate and acquired immunity.

Manipulating the oral immune response by development of drugs that inhibit adverse host reactions and promote beneficial effects might be of therapeutic or prophylactic importance in periodontal diseases.

This review intends to assess the importance of Toll-like receptors as main effectors of the innate immune response in the triggering, maintenance and progression of periodontal inflammation as well as of the involvement of synthetic molecules targeting TLR signalling networks in treating periodontal diseases.

2. Methodology

This chapter has been designed in order to assess the role of innate immune receptors, especially Toll-like receptors, as main effectors of the innate immune response triggered by various pathogens hosted in the subgingival film which are able to onset periodontal inflammation, as well as the involvement of synthetic molecules targeting TLR signalling pathways in treating periodontal diseases. Information processed has been sourced from the existing scientific literature and supplemented with our personal findings from experimental studies regarding TLR involvement in mediating innate immune response at oral mucosa level. We searched MEDLINE, Web of Science, SCOPUS, without language restriction, following terms „innate immunity" AND „periodontal inflammation" OR „periodontal disease" AND „TLR" OR „TLR therapeutic targets". Identification of specific literature also included manual search and screening of the citations of the relevant studies. The included studies were selected after reviewing the abstract and full-text for eligibility.

3. Oral mucosa cells and the innate immune response

The oral mucosa consists of a stratified oral epithelium formed by keratinocytes lining the inner connective tissue or *lamina propria* which has as main cells the fibroblasts and also proinflammatory cells originated in the bone marrow.

Three distinct phenotypes of oral mucosa are noted: lining, masticatory and specialised mucosa. The lining mucosa cover almost the entire mouth, excepting the rigid structures, such as the alveolar processes and the hard palate, which are covered by the masticatory mucosa, and the dorsal part of the tongue coated by the specialised mucosa [3]. The crevicular (CE) and junctional epithelium (JE) are the keystones for the antimicrobial barrier function of the oral mucosa. Compared to other types of epithelial cells, JE possesses fewer intercellular junctions, just desmosomes, and more intercellular spaces filled with gingival crevicular fluid (CF). Due to this histophysiology, JE allows the passage of CF, the carrier of inflammatory cells and soluble mediators, from the gingival connective tissue to the crevicular space. The changes of the dental biofilm and the metabolic products of bacteria trigger the synthesis of cytokines and increase the number of polymorphonuclear cells (PMNs) migrating to the initial site of inflammation. This early event, gingivitis, is followed by the appearance of other inflammatory cells (macrophages, lymphocytes, mononuclear and dendritic cells) and the persistence of inflammation of the teeth supporting tissues with progressive attachment loss and bone destruction, namely periodontitis [4]. The proinflammatory cells of the oral mucosa connective tissue are myeloid-originated immune cells such as monocytes, macrophages and dendritic cells which act as the first line of defence during infection, recognising, engulfing and killing bacteria, fungi or viruses. Recent data emphasises that it is not only the immune cells but also the fibroblasts and the keratinocytes that contribute to local immunity through the activation and modulation of specific immune receptors [5]. Fibroblasts activation triggered by the immune cells is involved in the remodelling of the extracellular matrix (ECM); moreover, under the stimulation of the endothelial cells derived signals, fibroblasts are able to differentiate into myofibroblasts important for wound healing of the masticatory mucosa [6]. Knowledge of how immune mechanisms and responses are controlled is essential for understanding the pathogenesis of periodontal inflammation. Bacteria are the most common pathogens in the case of gingivitis, followed by periodontitis, but both pathologies can also be caused by other pathogens like fungi, viruses or by metabolic imbalances. Until recently, innate and specific/adaptive immune responses had been arbitrarily proposed by immunologists as two distinct stages of the immunologic events. Later it was clarified that adaptive or acquired immune response evolved around innate immunity instead of replacing it. The development of acquired immunity is regulated through the activation of some myeloid and antigen presenting cells (APCs). Innate immunity should be considered as an immune system skill developed in order "to buy time" [7] until the acquired, more efficient host immune response, is primed. The immune system has a hierarchical organisation containing immune cells (monocytes, macrophages, neutrophils, dendritic cells (DCs), natural killer cells (NK), mast cells, eosinophils, basophils and newly identified innate lymphoid cells (ILCs), mucosal associated invariant T cells, $\gamma\delta$T cells) and humoral circulating components (complement proteins, cytokines and chemokines secreted by those cells, along with various antimicrobial peptides, AMPs) [2, 8–11]. All the cells already mentioned are able to sense the pathogens through PRRs and then develop the innate immune response [12]. A limited number of PRRs are able to recognise a large number of pathogens. PRRs detect and respond to conserved motifs originated in microorganisms and stress signals called PAMPS and DAMPS [1]. PAMPs are evolutionarily conserved structures shared among pathogens, but not present in eukaryotes, which confer specificity to the innate immune response. These include lipopolysaccharides, peptidoglycans, bacterial lipoproteins, DNA and double stranded RNA [7]. DAMPs are endogenous ligands derived from host cells (tumour cells, dying cells) or products released from cells in response to various signals which produce inflammation in the absence of infection. DAMPs are often created in environments of trauma, ischemia, or tissue damage involved in various diseases (cancer, autoimmune disease, and atherosclerosis) and do not require pathogens infection [1, 13]. Inside the more generic term microbial-associated molecular patterns (MAMPs), one could consider commensal-associated molecular patterns (CAMPs), as many microorganisms colonise the human body without causing disease [14]. PAMPs, MAMPs and DAMPs bind to PPRs which include mainly Toll-like receptors (TLRs), transmembrane C-type lectin-like receptors (CLRs), cytoplasmic NOD-like receptors (NLRs) and intracellular retinoic acid-inducible gene-I-like receptors (RLR) [13, 15]. PRR-ligand binding and their concomitant conformational changes prompt a cascade of downstream signalling that results in transcriptional and post-translational changes. Among these PRRs, TLRs have been studied most extensively.

4. Toll-like receptors: structure, ligands and signalling

TLRs, so called because they are similar to the product of the Toll gene identified in *Drosophila*, are the best characterised from all the classes of PRRs. Until now, ten human TLRs have been described, the first being reported 26 years ago by Nomura in 2004 [16] and called TLR1. TLRs are evolutionary conserved transmembrane glycoproteins that contain an extracellular (or intra-cytosolic for those intracellular TLRs expressed in endosomes) N-terminal leucin-rich-repeat (LRR) domain, a transmembrane domain and an intra-cytoplasmic Toll/IL-1R (TIR) domain. LRR is responsible for ligand recognition and binding while TIR domain for intracellular signal transfer [14]. It is generally accepted that most TLRs are localised to the cell surface (TLR1, TLR2, TLR4, TLR5, TLR6 and TLR10) and recognised extracellular microorganisms and ligands, while TLR3, TLR7, TLR8 and TLR9 are intracellular, hosted into the cytosolic endosomal compartment and recognised molecular patterns that have already passed the cell membrane [14]. Recently has been demonstrated that TLR2 and TLR4are also present inside some cells: DCs, monocytes, epithelial and endothelial cells [17, 18]. The cells expressing TLRs in humans and their ligands are listed in **Table 1**.

Toll-like receptor	Cells	Ligands
TLR 1	Neutrophils, monocytes/macrophages Myeloid and plasmacytoid dendritic cells* B lymphocytes Fibroblasts, Keratinocytes Endothelial cells	Triacyllipopeptides
TLR 2	Neutrophils, monocytes/macrophages Myeloid dendritic cells T lymphocytes Fibroblasts, Keratinocytes Endothelial cells	Lipoproteins Peptidoglycan Lipoteichoic acid Zymosan *P. gingivalis* LPS *C. ochracea* LPS
TLR 3	Myeloid dendritic cells B lymphocytes, Th1/Th2 lymphocytes Fibroblasts, Keratinocytes Endothelial cells	dsRNA, Polyinosine Polycytidilic acid
TLR 4	Neutrophils, monocytes/macrophages Myeloid dendritic cells Fibroblasts, Keratinocytes Endothelial cells	Most bacterial LPS
TLR 5	Neutrophils, monocytes/macrophages Myeloid dendritic cells Th1/Th2 lymphocytes Fibroblasts, Keratinocytes Endothelial cells	Flagellin

Toll-like receptor	Cells	Ligands
TLR 6	Neutrophils, monocytes/macrophages Myeloid and plasmacytoid dendritic cells B lymphocytes Fibroblasts, Keratinocytes Endothelial cells	Peptidoglycan Lipoteichoic acid Diacyllipopeptides Zymosan
TLR 7	Neutrophils, monocytes/macrophages Plasmacytoid dendritic cells B lymphocytes,Fibroblasts	Immunomodulatory drugs (imiquimod, resiquimod)
TLR 8	Neutrophils, monocytes/macrophages Myeloid dendritic cells Treg lymphocytes Fibroblasts	ssRNA Immunomodulatory drugs (imiquimod, resiquimod)
TLR 9	Neutrophils Plasmacytoid dendritic cells B lymphocytes, Th1/Th2 lymphocytes Fibroblasts, Keratinocytes Endothelial cells	Bacterial DNA Viral DNA CpG Oligodeoxynucleotide
TLR 10	Neutrophils Myeloid dendritic cells B lymphocytes Fibroblasts, Keratinocytes	Orphan receptor

**In human blood, two subpopulations of DCs precursors are present – myeloid or conventional and plasmacytoid - different in terms of cell phenotype and morphology, which express various TLRs. Plasmacytoid DCs recognise predominantly viral antigens through the activation of TLR7 and TLR9 [19, 20]. Myeloid or classical DCs recognise both bacterial and viral antigens [21, 22].*

Table 1.
Toll-like receptors expressing cells in humans and their ligands.

In physiologic conditions, the intracellular TLRs have no contact with host cells derived nucleic acids because they are sequestered in endosomes and no innate response is signalled against own nucleic acids. In some pathologic conditions, TLRs signal the synthesis of autoantibodies against host own nucleic acids, for example in rheumatoid polyarthritis, much evidence showing the link between rheumatoid arthritis and periodontal disease [23] which may suggest a similar expression of these receptors in the diseases having in common the destruction of hard tissues.

TLR 1, TLR2, TLR4, TLR5 and TLR6 recognise mainly unique bacterial products and not those produced by the host, which gives them the ability to differentiate microorganisms from the host and conveys some degree of specificity, making them the missing link between the innate and acquired immunity [24].

TLR2 and TLR4 are the most defined members of this family. TLR2 forms heterodimers with TLR1 and TLR6 and recognises peptidoglycans, lipopeptides and lipoproteins, while TLR4 is the acknowledged PRR for lipopolysaccharide (LPS) and Gram-negative bacteria. Published data is conflicting regarding the ability of TLR4 to recognise *Porphyromonas gingivalis* and *Escherichia coli* LPS, some authors considering that TLR4 is able to detect only *E. coli* product [25, 26]. TLR3 recognises double-stranded RNA (dsRNA), TLR7 and TLR8 are known to recognise single-stranded RNA (ssRNA). TLR5 detects bacterial flagellin and TLR9 recognises cytosine and guanine base-pairing of bacterial and viral DNA [3, 27, 28].

LRR domain of TLRs is involved in the recognition of various ligands. LRR ligand binding induces the formation of TLRs homodimers or heterodimers followed by a conformational change of the TIR domain which allows the interaction between TIRs of adjacent TLRs in order to bind an additional adapter protein essential to trigger the intracellular signal cascade generating chemokines, cytokines and AMP.

In the same cell, the activation of different TLRs induces various proinflammatory responses. For example, the interaction of TLR3 and TLR4 with LPS in DCs triggers the synthesis of IL-12, and respectively type 1 interferon [29].

The same TLR can trigger a different response depending on the upper intracellular adapter protein [30].

To date, two different pathways are recognised for the intracytoplasmic signalling cascade of TLRs: (i) the myeloid differentiation primary response protein 88 (MyD 88) dependent pathway – the most important – essential for the majority of TLR-mediated cell activation, and (ii) MyD88-independent pathway, after TLR3 and TLR4 stimulation takes place. Even if the cells are forced to react to an extensive number of PAMPs, only four adapter molecules have been identified for both pathways: MyD88, toll/interleukin-1 receptor domain-containing adapter protein (TIRAP), toll/interleukin-1 receptor domain-containing adapter-inducing interferon beta (TRIF) and toll/interleukin-1 receptor domain-containing adapter-inducing interferon beta-related adapter molecule (TRAM) [3, 7, 14, 29, 31].

MyD88-dependent signalling predominantly leads to nuclear factor-kB (NF-kB) activation while the TRIF-dependent pathway, MyD88-independent, leads to interferon-regulatory factor 3 (IRF3) and to a lesser extent to NF-kB activation [31]. NF-kB is a crucial transcription factor that promotes the expression of genes encoding proinflammatory and chemotactic cytokines, such as IL-1, IL-12, IFNγ, CXCL9, CXCL10, costimulatory molecules and other effectors [32–34]. Apart from NF-kB activation, TRIF-dependent pathway induces the expression of type I interferons, mainly IFNβ [31, 35].

5. Toll-like receptors in periodontal diseases

Both in gingivitis and periodontitis a plethora of bacterial germs are accumulated in the gingival mucosa around the tooth, particularly in the gingival crevice [29]. More than 600 species populate the oral cavity [36, 37] with a clearest distinction between those characteristic of shedding epithelia (oral mucosa) and non-shedding surfaces - the tooth biofilm. The complex studies of oral microbiota have demonstrated a conspicuous change of the oral bacterial populations before and during the periodontal disease, making possible the definition of the 'red complex bacteria' including *Porphyromonas gingivalis, Tannerella forsythia* and *Treponema denticola* [38–40]. Recent investigations partially disagree with this paradigm and collectively suggest that the pathogenesis of periodontitis involves not only a polymicrobial synergy and a dysbiosis - the PSD model, but also a host susceptibility to chronic inflammatory disorders leading to an unbalanced immune response, which may trigger the limited success of the antimicrobial treatment [40].

Oral tissues homeostasis involves the balance between the oral mucosa with its immunocompetent cells and the extreme vast oral microbiota. In this paper we do not intend to characterise the oral microbiota but the innate immune response of the oral structures to various germ triggers of inflammatory periodontal inflammation.

Regarding the development of dental plaque two main events imply the importance of the innate immune response. On one hand, gingivitis does not necessarily lead to periodontitis, which suggests that, despite massive dental plaque accumulation, stable gingival inflammation may represent a protective host response [41]. On the other hand, in cases in which gingivitis evolves to periodontitis, plaque accumulation induces the development of a dysbiotic, inflammophilic microbiota. Each of these events depends, in great part, on host ability to control the resolution of the inflammatory processes [40].

Due to the presence of a constantly large number of microorganisms in the oral cavity, TLR expression is essential for the maintenance of oral tissue immune homeostasis. *Porphyromonas gingivalis* (*P. gingivalis*) has recently been described as a" corrupter" of the innate immunity manipulating the host response rather than inducing by itself a chronic inflammation, being a low abundance constituent in rodent and also in human periodontitis associated biofilm [42, 43]. Such a germ is called a"keystone germ" able to impair host defence in order to compromise the homeostasis between the commensal microbiota and the host immune response. Under the influence of a keystone germs, the commensal bacteria become pathobionts, normally harmless symbionts that can become pathogenic under certain environmental conditions. Actually, no bone loss is effective in periodontitis induced by *P. gingivalis* in the absence of commensal microbiota. Even incomplete, an explanation of the corruption effect on TLR innate immune system by the commensal germs could be the observation that commensals and symbionts share similar MAMPs (LPS, peptidoglycans, lipoproteins) with pathogens, so they could induce PRRs activation [44].

In the oral mucosa, TLRs are predominantly expressed in neutrophils, monocytes, macrophages, and equally important DCs. Albeit the macrophages and DCs represent"professional APCs", the first cells responding to PAMPs are the epithelial cells from the oral mucosa, precisely the crevicular lining cells. As APCs, DCs and macrophages are responsible for the presentation of the antigen fragments together with the MHC class II to T cells in order to induce a costimulatory response.

Because TLRs are present in cells from all the structures of the oral mucosa either directly related to the immune local defence or not and their activation leads to redundant local inflammatory reactions, we intend to use a mechanistic approach to their effects in periodontal disease.

5.1 TLR signalling in the oral epithelium

Although the expression of mRNAs for TLR1 to TLR9 has been detected in the oral epithelial cells, the immunolocalisation of the corresponding proteins was variable. Immunohistochemical studies revealed that TLR1 to TLR9 are differentially expressed in the epithelial layers and connective tissue of the gingival samples collected from patients with periodontitis and healthy subjects [45, 46]. Increased TLRs expression towards the basal layer of the epithelium and the connective tissue in samples with periodontitis sustains their involvement in the pathogenesis of this disease. The percentage of TLR4 positive cells was higher in the spinous layer keratinocytes of the healthy tissues in contrast to the periodontitis samples which revealed higher expression in the basal keratinocytes.

TLR2 and TLR4 are the most studied receptors in relation to periodontal tissues. Mori et al. studied the immunohistochemical expression of TLR2, TLR4 and CD14 in samples of oral mucosa classified according to the degree of inflammation. They found that the ratio of TLR4 positive cells was higher in samples from the more severe inflamed tissue and that of TLR2 positive cells was the highest in the connective tissue subjacent to pocket epithelium of the severe inflamed group [47]. Becerik and co-workers reported the same expression of TLR4 in tissue excised from periodontitis sites [48]. Depending on the state of inflammation, TLR2 is highly expressed in the cells of the gingival basal layer and lower reaction was observed in cells of the superficial layers more exposed to pathogens [33, 45]. They presume this expression as a strategy of TLR2 to recognise the pathogens only when they invade the superficial layers of the oral epithelium in order to limit the overexpression of the proinflammatory cytokines and to maintain the oral tissue homeostasis. In bacterial periodontitis, TLR4 expression in gingival cells decreased in order to minimise the damage of oral tissues and bone [49]. This observation is in accordance with that reported by [50] regarding the decreased number of DCs in the oral epithelium of periodontitis samples compared to non-inflamed mucosa or gingivitis.

We performed an immunohistochemical study for TLR2 and TLR4 expression on samples collected from patients with various degree of gingival inflammation. In samples with gingivitis, we observed that TLR2 is expressed evenly in almost all layers of the gingival epithelium except in the superficial layer (**Figure 1a,b**). In the basal and parabasal layers, we noticed TLR2 positivity in dendritic extensions possibly belonging to Langerhans cells, in addition to an inconstantly positive reaction in keratinocytes (**Figure 1c**). Regarding TLR4 expression, we observed a decrease of positivity in the epithelium from the superficial layers to the basal one (**Figure 1d**). In the connective tissue, we noticed more TLR2 positive proinflammatory cells than TLR4 positive (unpublished data). In periodontitis samples, the immunohistochemical reaction for TLR2 in the epithelium was more intense than in gingivitis, TLR2

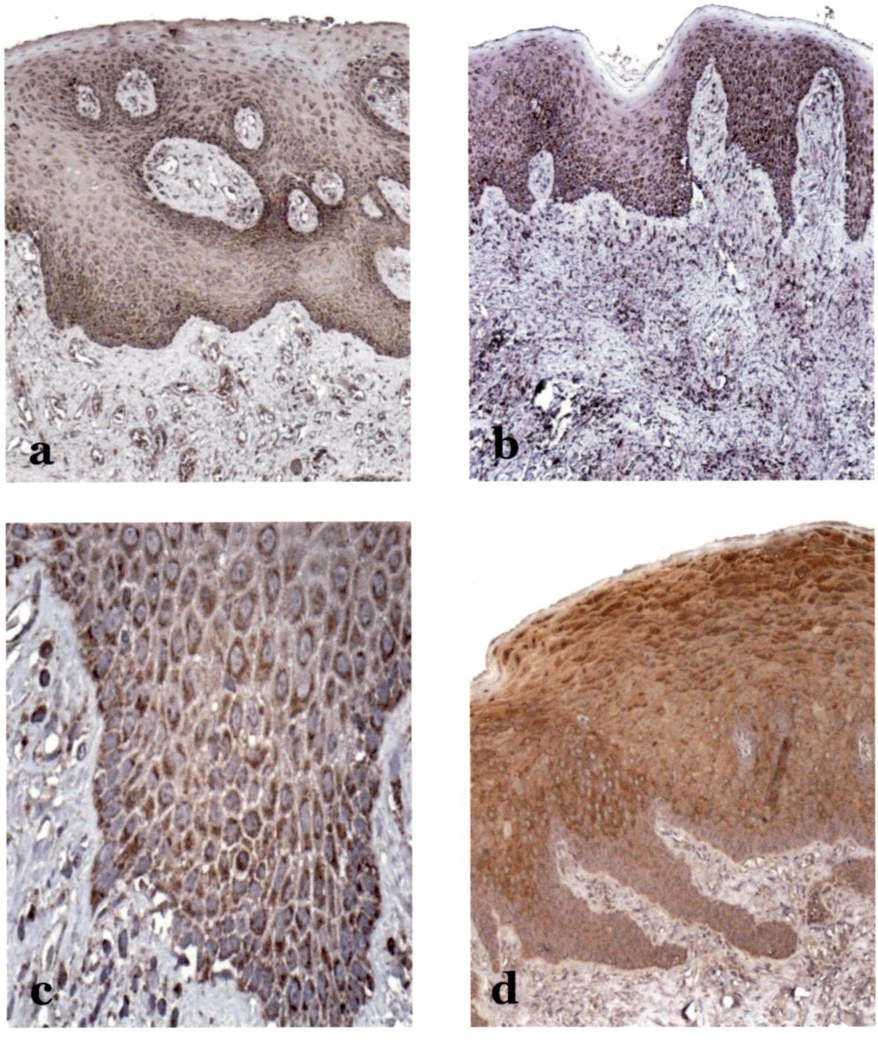

Figure 1.
TLR2 and TLR4 expression in gingivitis. (a) TLR2 positive keratinocytes into the basal and parabasal layers of the gingival epithelium; (b) Same positive reaction in the epithelium and also numerous TLR2 positive cells in the connective tissue, mainly in the vessel's walls; (c) TLR2 positivity in non-keratinocyte cells; (d) Inconstant intensity for TLR4 immune reaction in the epithelium.

being highly expressed in the basal layer (**Figure 2a**). In the connective tissue we noticed faint positivity in fibroblasts and some endothelial cells (**Figure 2b**). Cells from the perivascular concentrated lymphoplasmacytic infiltrate were intensely positive for TLR2. Regarding TLR4 expression, we noticed more intense positive cells in the epithelial spinous layer than in the superficial and basal ones. In the connective tissue, TLR4-positive fibroblasts were increased in number and proinflammatory cells showed discrete positivity (**Figure 2c**).

For TLR7 and TLR8 expression a comparable distribution between healthy and diseased oral tissues was noticed [14].

The antimicrobial effects induced by the activation of TLR2-TLR5 and TLR9 in the oral mucosa is also provided by the secretion of antimicrobial substances, more important being the α-, β-, and θ-defensins [14]. Defensins represent a class of cationic antimicrobial peptides secreted by the epithelial cells and neutrophils to play pivotal roles in innate and adaptive immunity, as well as roles in non-immunological processes. They have evolved to be highly efficient in their antimicrobial responses

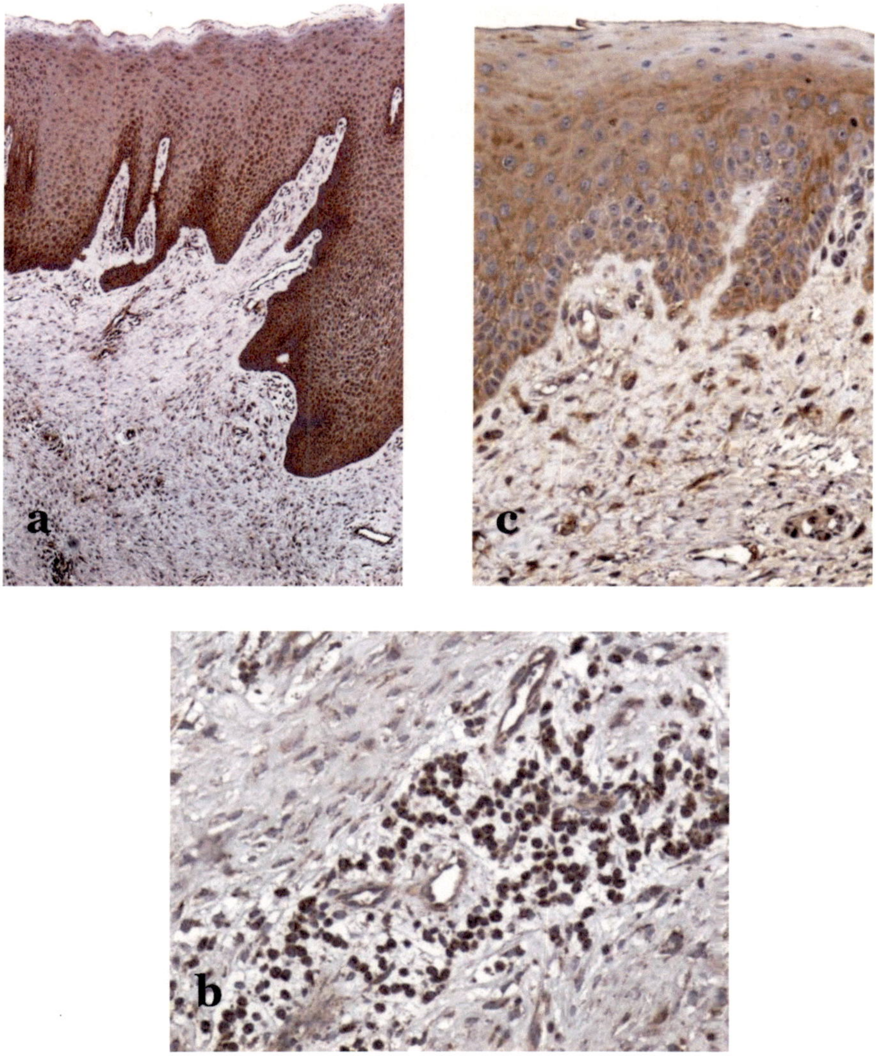

Figure 2.
TLR2 and TLR4 expression in periodontitis (a) Intense TLR2 positive reaction in the epithelial basal layer; (b) TLR2 positive cells spread in the lamina propria and proinflammatory cells concentrated in the proximity of vessels; (c) Different intensity of TLR 4 immune reaction through the keratinocyte layer. Fibroblasts show intense positivity in the superficial lamina propria. Vessels were was also TLR4 positive

to a vast array of pathogens [51]. mRNAs for β-defensins and their protein products were identified in the human oral epithelium [52].

Reported data sustains that TLR-induced expression of β-defensins is followed by two cellular events: (i) in a positive feedback mechanism, β-defensins themselves stimulate TLR signalling, acting as an epithelial immune inducer and (ii) they contribute to the recruitment/activation of several professional APCs, i.e. DCs and monocytes [52, 53].

5.2 TLR signalling beyond the basal membrane of the oral epithelium

Because the innate immune response is limited, slow and nonspecific for the antimicrobial defence, it is necessary to activate the specific immune response represented by B and T lymphocytes that invade the oral tissues a few days after their activation under DCs stimulation. In the oral epithelium, once activated by various stimuli, including TLR ligands, DCs (also called Langerhans cells by the analogy with those in the epidermis) mature, acquire high phagocytic capacity, express the chemokine receptor 7 (CCR7) and become mobiles. Through the *lamina propria*, they migrate to the neighbouring lymph node where they activate CD4 + T cells (T helper, Th) [54] being the most potent APCs activating naïve T cells and consequently the main messengers between innate and adaptive immune system. Under DCs instructions, CD4 + Th differentiate into various subtypes: Th1, Th2, Th17, T regulatory cells (Treg) [54]. The action of DCs on T lymphocytes is a complex process triggered by a various constellation of cytokines dependent on tissue of origin and DCs maturation state [55]. There is little information regarding the subtypes of DCs identified in the *lamina propria* of oral mucosa in humans. DCs have the ability to decide whether or not to respond and what kind of immune response to develop against a particular pathogen or a group of microorganisms. They are activated not only by germs but also by non-immune cells - fibroblasts and keratinocytes, that produce proinflammatory cytokines as a result of exposure to various pathogens. These substances are able to induce different responses in DCs which in turn are provided with the ability to modulate downstream the adaptive immune response.

The number of DCs in gingival mucosa is related to the topographic area and to the degree of inflammation. In normal human mucosa their number in the sulcular epithelium seems to increase with the accumulation of dental plaque [50, 56, 57]. In a model of human gingivitis, some authors showed that the number of DCs decreased by day 21st of inflammation [58]. This variation of incidence is in accordance with the observation that DCs could have a stimulating inflammatory effect in gingival inflammation by the induction of Th1 or Th17 response through IL-12 and IFN ɣ [59] and also a protective effect, cushioning the immune response by stimulating Treg through IL-10 and TGF- βsecretion [20, 60].

A lower number of LCs or a reduced level of CD1a produced by LCs were found in the epithelium during chronic periodontitis compared to gingivitis [59, 61, 62] suggesting that LCs leave the oral epithelium as the inflammation progresses. Other authors did not notice any difference between healthy and inflamed gingiva in periodontitis, or even reported an increased number of DCs [63, 64]. It is difficult to monitor the chronological overlap between the disappearance of LCs and the degree of inflammation and one can suspect that the development of inflammation is due to the low number of DCs. In fact, a link between the high incidence of periodontitis in elderly and the decreased number of DCs in these subjects was highlighted [65].

Chemokines and cytokines produced by DCs in response to their activation through the interaction with pathogens, such as *P. gingivalis*, can attract neutrophils and monocytes to the site of inflammation [20].

DOI: http://dx.doi.org/10.5772/intechopen.96801

Neutrophils and monocytes are the main blood innate immune cells and they pass through the capillary wall into the *lamina propria* of the oral mucosa. IL-8 secreted by the epithelial cells stimulates through TLR4 the adhesion of endothelial cells lining the vessels to monocytes by an increased expression of adhesion molecules E-selectin, Intercellular Adhesion Molecule-1 (ICAM-1) and Vascular Cell Adhesion Molecule-1 (VCAM-1) [66]. Once in the tissue, the monocytes mature as macrophages or activated macrophages. Depending on the activating substances, the macrophages are phenotypically polarised: M1 macrophages are the classic macrophagic cell, activated by IFN-ɣ and LPS, while the M2 macrophage phenotype is involved in the resolution of inflammation and fibrosis [29].

Both neutrophils and macrophages – phagocytic cells from a myeloid lineage - are considered to represent the first line of defence against microbial pathogens. Neutrophils express TLR 1, 2, 4-10 and macrophages TLR 1, 2, 4-8 (see **Table 1**). When stimulated via TLR, neutrophils display an increased chemotaxis and synthesis of defensins, proinflammatory cytokines (IL-1, IL-6, TNF-α) [67]. All these substances are involved in tissue destruction and stimulation of bone resorption. Noteworthy, neutrophils migration into JE was dependent of commensal colonisation and MYD 88 activation pathway [68, 69]. Chang et al. demonstrated that TLR2 and TLR4 are not required for promoting neutrophil trafficking into JE but may substantially contribute to shape the composition of microbiota which may modulate neutrophil homeostasis. Direct recognition of bacteria by TLR2 and TLR4 is not necessary for neutrophil migration into the gingival sulcus [70].

When exposed to PAMPS, monocytes can differentiate into osteoclasts upon direct stimulation of LPS by the help of RANKL [71, 72] and they also produce proinflammatory cytokines. In periodontitis, mature osteoclasts derived from DCs and monocytes are molecularly identical despite the fact that fewer genes must be activated when osteoclasts are formed from DCs than from monocyte precursors [73].

Two possibilities of evolution can be described for gingival inflammation: (i) the return to tissue homeostasis after an acute inflammation, as a protective response to bacterial biofilm, which is an active sequence of events and (ii) the persistence of inflammation leading to activation of gingival fibroblasts and myofibroblasts, in case of failure of resolution pathways, with destruction of ECM and bone, followed by scar formation and fibrosis, preventing the return of tissue homeostasis [74]. Various antibodies could be used to identify the fibroblasts phenotype: vimentin, α-SMA and S100-A4 (FSP1). There is a marked phenotypic heterogeneity of fibroblasts in gingival mucosa, as myofibroblasts are least represented and the cells positive for FSP1 are most commonly present [75]. Fibroblasts are intimately linked with the immune innate system. Uehara and Takada indicated that almost all TLRs from gingival fibroblasts are functionally involved in periodontal inflammatory reactions acting mainly by the MYD88 dependent pathway [5]. Once stimulated by PAMPs, fibroblasts produce proinflammatory cytokines leading directly to periodontal tissue destruction and bone resorption. Fibroblasts involvement in gingival inflammation has been intensively studied in connection to *P. gingivalis* infection. LPS from *P. gingivalis* activates TLRs from gingival fibroblasts and the synthesis of MMP1 and MMP3 to degrade ECM. MMPs in turn induce the expression of IL-1β, IL-6, IL-8 and MCP1 [6] which upregulate the inflammatory response in tissue-dependent manner. When comparing human periodontal ligament fibroblasts with human gingival fibroblasts isolated from the same donor to examine IL-8 responses of the cells to some germs and the possible involvement of the CD14/TLR system, the authors found that gingival fibroblasts strongly expressed CD14 mRNA and CD14 protein while periodontal ligament fibroblasts showed lower levels of expression in both respects [76]. Both types of fibroblasts expressed mRNA of

TLR2, TLR4, MD2 and MyD88, with TLR2 expression more intense in cells from the periodontal ligament [76]. Moreover, gingival fibroblasts exhibited a stronger IL-8 response than those from the periodontal ligament to LPS. The ability of periodontal fibroblasts to develop an adequate secondary immune response to *P. gingivalis* LPS could be compromised with persistence of inflammation.

6. Nucleotide-binding oligomerisation domain (NOD)-like receptors signalling

The NOD-like (NLR) family of innate intracellular receptors detects several PAMPs and endogenous molecules. In humans, this family contains ~20 members classified into five different subfamilies according to their structure: (i) NLRA which has an acidic transactivation domain, (ii) NLRB - with a baculovirus inhibitor of apoptosis protein repeat, (iii) NLRC – contains a CARD domain and includes NOD1 and NOD2, (iv) NLRP – which as a pyrin domain and responds to multiple stimuli forming a multiprotein complex termed NALP – inflammasome, and the last (v) NLRX, containing an uncharacterized domain [31, 77, 78]. A number of putative ligands of NLRs have been reported, but the field of NLRs ligand identification is still open. It is unclear whether NLRs, as well as TLRs, are able to interact directly through the LRR domain with their ligands [79]. NODs are cytosolic PRRs that bind to peptidoglycan from bacterial cell wall. NOD1 and NOD2 are present more or less in the same immune cells as TLR: NOD1 on human mononuclear cells, macrophages, epithelial cells, including those from oral epithelium, and dendritic cells, while NOD2 is present mostly on phagocytic cells: macrophages, DCs, neutrophils [80, 81] and Paneth cells of the small intestine [82–84]. NOD1 is involved in recognising cell wall compounds from Gram-negative bacteria, while NOD2 can sense both Gram-positive and Gram-negative bacterial cell wall components [82, 85]. NOD1 plays an essential role in innate immune response, its downstream signalling inducing the production of proinflammatory cytokines (IL-6, IL-8, TNF-α, hBD-2) and chemokines, as well as compounds with immunoregulatory and antimicrobial properties (IFN-γ, hBD-1).

The inflammasome comprises proteins that are assembled by intracytoplasmic PRRs. A multitude of inflammasomes exist and these can be activated through various mechanisms in order to secrete proinflammatory cytokines [86]. Once activated by PAMPs or DAMPs, the NLRPs undergo conformational changes that trigger the activation of caspase-1. Afterwards, the maturation of proinflammatory cytokines, such as IL-1β and IL-18, to their active forms follows and finally results in inflammation and pyroptosis, a cellular event confirmed in periodontal inflammation [87, 88]. Pyroptosis is a proinflammatory programmed cell death pathway uniquely dependent on caspase-1 [89]. The mechanism and outcome of pyroptosis are different from those of apoptosis which actively inhibits inflammation.

Fourteen members of the NLRP subfamily are described [90]. Among these, expression NLRP2 inflammasome was reported to be decreased in gingival epithelia infected by *P. gingivalis* [91]. NLRP1 and NLRP3 are proposed to be involved in inflammasome function in addition to the cytoplasmic receptor absent in melanoma 2 (AIM2) [92]. AIM2 is the first non-NLR family member that was identified to mediate inflammasome assembly and activate the caspase-1 pathway [93] having mainly cytosolic dsDNA from viruses, bacteria or the host as ligands. NLRP1, NLRP3 and AIM2 may exhibit inflammasome activity in diseases such as type 2 diabetes, essential hypertension or rheumatoid arthritis [88].

It is confirmed that the expression level of the inflammasome changes as the inflammation destroys the gingival tissues [91, 94]. In an immunohistochemical study, Xue et al. described a dissimilar expression pattern of NLRP1, NLRP3 and AIM2 in chronic and aggressive periodontitis, demonstrating their involvement in the pathogenesis of periodontal diseases to different degrees [88]. NLRP3 was significantly higher in chronic periodontitis and more expressed in the gingival epithelium than in *lamina propria* both in periodontitis and gingivitis The intensity was gradually weaker from the top to the basal membrane in chronic periodontitis and opposite in aggressive periodontitis, which strengthens the idea that the bacteria outside the gingiva are more important in the pathogenesis of gingivitis when in aggressive periodontitis the host factor may be more importantly involved [88]. NLRP1 seems not to be an important biomarker for distinguishing gingivitis, aggressive and chronic periodontitis, because they observed that NLRP1 was barely expressed in gingival tissues in both conditions.

7. Therapeutic perspectives of TLR targeting in periodontal inflammation

Usual practical approaches to reduce bacterial levels to proportions manageable by the host innate immune system and limit the aggression of oral pathogens on periodontal tissues (scaling, root planning and meticulous oral hygiene techniques) [95] are often inefficient and for this reason adjunctive therapeutic strategies have been proposed in order to modulate host response.

Since their discovery, TLRs have emerged as pivotal mediators of innate host immune and inflammatory response. Due to their role in the recognition of PAMPS and DAMPS of various origins and the triggering of a proinflammatory response, TLR-signalling is regarded as a novel therapeutic target. That is why research was conducted to develop drugs that exploit TLRs signalling in immune therapy, drugs which are already tried to treat diseases, such as asthma and chronic obstructive pulmonary disease [96], AIDS [97], hepatitis B [98, 99], cancer [100, 101].

To date, several directions for targeting TLR-signalling pathways are discussed:

- Negative regulation for prevention of aberrant activation of TLRs;
- Use of synthetic substitutes;
- TLR as vaccine adjuvants;
- TLR agonists;
- TLR antagonists [102].

Despite the potential of TLRs to activate the synthesis of protective molecules against infection, they can also induce serious immunopathological reactions in case of overstimulation or insufficient control due to the limited action of some negative regulators. An increased number of negative regulators able to dampen the degree and duration of TLR-mediated inflammatory host response were proposed.

Negative regulation of TLR signalling can be exerted extracellularly (inhibition of receptor function) or intracellularly (inhibition of downstream signalling).

Negative regulation occurs through different mechanisms:

- Soluble decoy TLRs, for example isoforms of TLR4, induced by various stimuli are able to block TLRs signalling and production of corresponding cytokines and chemokines [103];
- Degradation of signal proteins [104];
- Transcriptional regulation. Several miRNAs are reported to be essential modulators of immune pathways because they target adaptor molecules and their expression varies following TLR activation [104].

Negative regulators fail to control TLRs signalling because requiring a combination of effects, their loss leads to hyperactivation and pathogens develop strategies to evade TLR signalling [104]. TLRs may be novel therapeutic targets in periodontitis since manipulation of their signalling pathways contribute to the control of infection and inflammation and TLR agonists could be tested as vaccine adjuvants in treating periodontal inflammation [105].

Vaccine adjuvants exert their action by increasing antigen delivery to APCs, activating them to produce cytokines and by triggering T lymphocytes response [102, 106]. TLRs can function as adjuvant receptors for the recognition of certain antigens produced by microorganisms, the stimulation and maturation of APCs and the alerting of the immune system [24].

TLR agonists, similar but less toxic than PAMPS, are able to cause DCs maturation [102]. They are small molecules that mimic natural TLR ligands and could have improved pharmacological effects.

TLRs agonists are already clinically tested as vaccine adjuvants for cancer, allergic and infectious diseases [107].

8. Conclusion

Innate immune receptors are critical in maintaining periodontal health as well as in the progression of gingival inflammation by acting on the commensal microbiome and as a link to the activation of adaptive immunity. Due to the fact that TLRs are important in preserving the periodontium state in healthy conditions and TLR-inflammation is responsible for the destructive host reactions in periodontal diseases, the development of drugs that target TLR signalling and promote beneficial local effects would be of great success in such diseases.

Conflict of interest

None.

Author details

Ana Marina Andrei[1], Elena Cristina Andrei[2], Elena Camelia Stănciulescu[1], Mihaela Cezarina Mehedinți[3], Mihaela Jana Țuculină[4], Ileana Monica Baniță[2]*, Sandra Alice Buteică[5] and Cătălina Gabriela Pisoschi[1]

1 Department of Pharmaceutical Biochemistry, Faculty of Pharmacy, University of Medicine and Pharmacy, Craiova, Romania

2 Department of Histology, Faculty of Dentistry, University of Medicine and Pharmacy, Craiova, Romania

3 Department of Histology, Faculty of Medicine and Pharmacy, University "Dunarea de Jos", Galati, Romania

4 Department of Conservative and Restorative Odontotherapy, Faculty of Dentistry, University of Medicine and Pharmacy, Craiova, Romania

5 Department of Therapeutic Chemistry, Faculty of Pharmacy, University of Medicine and Pharmacy, Craiova, Romania

*Address all correspondence to: monica.banita@yahoo.com

References

[1] Tang D, Kang R, Coyne CB, Zeh HJ, Lotze MT. PAMPs and DAMPs: signal 0s that spur autophagy and immunity. Immunological Reviews. 2012 Sep;249(1):158-175. DOI: 10.1111/j.1600-065X.2012.01146.x

[2] Vijay K. Toll-like receptors in immunity and inflammatory diseases: Past, present, and future. International Immunopharmacology. 2018; 59: 391-412. DOI: 10.1016/j.intimp.2018.03.002

[3] Groeger S, Meyle J. Oral Mucosal Epithelial Cells. Frontiers in Immunology. 2019;10:208. DOI: 10.3389/fimmu.2019.00208

[4] Flemmig TF. Periodontitis. Annals of Periodontology. 1999; 4:32-38. DOI: 10.1902/annals.1999.4.1.32

[5] Uehara A, Takada H. Functional TLRs and NODs in human gingival fibroblasts. Journal of Dental Research. 2007;86(3):249-254. DOI: 10.1177/154405910708600310

[6] Alfonso García SL, Parada-Sanchez MT, Arboleda Toro T. The phenotype of gingival fibroblasts and their potential use in advanced therapies. European Journal of Cell Biology. 2020;99:151123. DOI:10.1016/j.ejcb.2020.151123

[7] Hans M, Hans VM. Toll-like receptors and their dual role in periodontitis: a review. Journal of Oral Science. 2011;53(3):263-271. DOI: 10.2334/josnusd.53.263

[8] Silva MT. When two is better than one: macrophages and neutrophils work in concert in innate immunity as complementary and cooperative partners of a myeloid phagocyte system. Journal of Leukocyte Biology. 2010;87(1):93-106. DOI:10.1189/jlb.0809549

[9] Wiesner J, Vilcinskas A. Antimicrobial peptides: the ancient arm of the human immune system. Virulence. 2010;1(5):440-464. DOI: 10.4161/viru.1.5.12983.

[10] Morgan BP, Harris CL. Complement, a target for therapy in inflammatory and degenerative diseases. Nature Reviews Drug Discovery. 2015;14(12):857-877. DOI: 10.1038/nrd4657

[11] de Oliveira S, Rosowski EE, Huttenlocher A. Neutrophil migration in infection and wound repair: going forward in reverse. Nature Reviews Immunology. 2016;16(6):378-391. DOI: 10.1038/nri.2016.49

[12] Takeuchi O, Akira S. Pattern recognition receptors and inflammation. Cell. 2010;140(6):805-820. DOI: 10.1016/j.cell.2010.01.022

[13] Schaefer L. Complexity of danger: the diverse nature of damage-associated molecular patterns. Journal of Biological Chemistry. 2014;289(51):35237-35245. DOI: 10.1074/jbc.R114.61930

[14] McClure R, Massari P. TLR-Dependent Human Mucosal Epithelial Cell Responses to Microbial Pathogens. Frontiers in Immunology. 2014; 5: 386. DOI: 10.3389/fimmu.2014.00386. eCollection 2014

[15] Mogensen TH. Pathogen Recognition and Inflammatory Signaling in Innate Immune Defenses. Clinical Microbiology Reviews. 2009; 22(2): 240-273. DOI: 10.1128/CMR.00046-08

[16] Nomura N, Miyajima N, Sazuka T, Tanaka A, Kawarabayasi Y, Sato S, Nagase T, Seki N, Ishikawa K, Tabata S. Prediction of the coding sequences of unidentified human genes. I. The coding sequences of 40 new genes (KIAA0001-KIAA0040) deduced by analysis of

randomly sampled cDNA clones from human immature myeloid cell line KG-1. DNA Research. 1994;1:27-35. DOI: 10.1093/dnares/1.1.47

[17] Hornef MW, Normark BH, Vandewalle A, Normark S. Intracellular recognition of lipopolysaccharide by toll-like receptor 4 in intestinal epithelial cells. Journal of Experimental Medicine. 2003;198(8):1225-1235. DOI: 10.1084/jem.20022194

[18] Uronen-Hansson H, Allen J, Osman M, Squires G, Klein N, Callard RE. Toll-like receptor 2 (TLR2) and TLR4 are present inside human dendritic cells, associated with microtubules and the Golgi apparatus but are not detectable on the cell surface: integrity of microtubules is required for interleukin-12 production in response to internalised bacteria. Immunology. 2004;111(2):173-178. DOI: 10.1111/j.0019-2805.2003.01803.x

[19] Swiecki M, Colonna M. The multifaceted biology of plasmacytoid dendritic cells. Nature Reviews Immunology. 2015;15(8):471-485. DOI: 10.1038/nri3865

[20] Song L, Dong G, Guo L, Graves DT. The function of dendritic cells in modulating the host response. Mol Oral Microbiol. 2018; 33(1): 13-21. DOI: 10.1111/omi.12195

[21] Steinman RM, Inaba K. Myeloid dendritic cells. Journal of Leukocyte Biology. 1999;66(2):205-208. DOI: 10.1002/jlb.66.2.205

[22] MacDonald KP, Munster DJ, Clark GJ, Dzionek A, Schmitz J, Hart DN. Characterization of human blood dendritic cell subsets. Blood. 2002;100(13):4512-4520. DOI: 10.1182/blood-2001-11-0097

[23] Bingham CO 3rd, Moni M. Periodontal disease and rheumatoid arthritis: the evidence accumulates for complex pathobiologic interactions. Current Opinion in Rheumatology. 2013;25(3):345-353. DOI: 10.1097/BOR.0b013e32835fb8ec

[24] Iwasaki A, Medzhitov R. Toll-like receptor control of the adaptive immune responses. Nature Immunology. 2004;5:987-995. DOI:10.1038/ni1112

[25] Pulendran B, Kumar P, Cutler CW, Mohamadzadeh M, Van Dyke T, Banchereau J. Lipopolysaccharides from distinct pathogens induce different classes of immune responses in vivo. Journal of Immunology. 2001;167: 5067–5076. DOI: 10.4049/jimmunol.167.9.5067

[26] Jotwani R, Pulendran B, Agrawal S, Cutler CW. Human dendritic cells respond to Porphyromonas gingivalis LPS by promoting a Th2 effector response *in vitro*. European Journal of Immunology. 2003;33(11):2980-2986. DOI: 10.1002/eji.200324392

[27] Bauer S, Kirschning CJ, Häcker H, Redecke V, Hausmann S, Akira S, Wagner H, Lipford GB. Human TLR9 confers responsiveness to bacterial DNA via species-specific CpG motif recognition. Proceedings of the National Academy of Sciences of the United States of America. 2001;98(16):9237-9242. DOI: 10.1073/pnas.161293498

[28] Hayashi F, Smith KD, Ozinsky A, Hawn TR, Yi EC, Goodlett DR, Eng JK, Akira S, Underhill DM, Aderem A. The innate immune response to bacterial flagellin is mediated by Toll-like receptor 5. Nature. 2001;410(6832):1099-1103. DOI: 10.1038/35074106

[29] Cekici A, Kantarci A, Hasturk H, Van Dyke TE. Inflammatory and immune pathways in the pathogenesis of periodontal disease. Periodontology 2000.2014; 64(1):57-80. DOI: 10.1111/prd.12002

[30] Cook DN, Pisetsky DS, Schwartz DA. Toll-like receptors in the

pathogenesis of human disease. Nature Immunology. 2004;5:975-979. DOI: 10.1038/ni1116

[31] Oviedo-Boyso J, Bravo-Patiño A, Baizabal-Aguirre VM. Collaborative action of Toll-like and NOD-like receptors as modulators of the inflammatory response to pathogenic bacteria. Mediators of Inflammation. 2014;2014:432785. DOI: 10.1155/2014/432785

[32] Lebre MC, van der Aar AMG, van Baarsen L, van Capel TMM, Schuitemaker JHN, Kapsenberg ML, de Jong EC. Human keratinocytes express functional Toll-like receptor 3, 4, 5, and 9. Journal of Investigative Dermatology. 2007;127(2):331-341. DOI: 10.1038/sj.jid.5700530

[33] Semlali A, Witoled C, Alanazi M, Rouabhia M. Whole cigarette smoke increased the expression of TLRs, HBDs, and proinflammory cytokines by human gingival epithelial cells through different signaling pathways. PLoS One. 2012;7(12):e52614. DOI: 10.1371/journal.pone.0052614

[34] Jaitley S, Saraswathi T R. Pathophysiology of Langerhans cells. Journal of Oral Maxillofacial Pathology. 2012;16:239-244. DOI: 10.4103/0973-029X.99077

[35] Kawai T, Akira S. TLR signaling. Cell Death and Differentiation. 2006;13(5):816-825. DOI: 10.1038/sj.cdd.4401850

[36] Dewhirst FE, Chen T, Izard J, Paster BJ, Tanner ACR, Yu WH, Lakshmanan A, Wade WG. The human oral microbiome. Journal of Bacteriology. 2010;192(19):5002-5017. DOI: 10.1128/JB.00542-10

[37] Moutsopoulos NM, Konkel JE. Tissue-Specific Immunity at the Oral Mucosal Barrier. Trends in Immunology. 2018;39(4):276-287. DOI: 10.1016/j.it.2017.08.005

[38] Darveau RP, Hajishengallis G, Curtis MA. Porphyromonas gingivalis as a Potential Community Activist for Disease. Journal of Dental Research. 2012;91(9):816-820. DOI: 10.1177/0022034512453589

[39] Jiao Y, Hasegawa M, Inohara N. Emerging roles of immunostimulatory oral bacteria in periodontitis development. Trends in Microbiology. 2014;22(3):157-163. DOI: 10.1016/j.tim.2013.12.005

[40] Hajishengallis G. Immunomicrobial pathogenesis of periodontitis: keystones, pathobionts, and host response. Trends in Immunology. 2014;35(1):3-11. DOI: 10.1016/j.it.2013.09.001

[41] Graves DT, Oates T, Garlet GP. Review of osteoimmunology and the host response in endodontic and periodontal lesions. Journal of Oral Microbiology. 201;3. DOI: 10.3402/jom.v3i0.5304

[42] Hajishengallis G, Liang S, Payne MA, Hashim A, Jotwani R, Eskan MA, McIntosh ML, Alsam A, Kirkwood KL, Lambris JD, Darveau RP, Curtis MA. Low-abundance biofilm species orchestrates inflammatory periodontal disease through the commensal microbiota and complement. Cell Host Microbe. 2011;10(5):497-506. DOI: 10.1016/j.chom.2011.10.006

[43] Abusleme L, Dupuy AK, Dutzan N, Silva N, Burleson JA, Strausbaugh LD, Gamonal J, Diaz PI. The subgingival microbiome in health and periodontitis and its relationship with community biomass and inflammation. ISME Journal. 2013;7(5):1016-1025. DOI: 10.1038/ismej.2012.174

[44] Hajishengallis G, Darveau RP, Curtis MA. The keystone-pathogen hypothesis. Nature Reviews Microbiology. 2012;10(10):717-725. DOI: 10.1038/nrmicro2873

[45] Beklen A, Hukkanen M, Richardson R, Konttinen YT. Immunohistochemical localization of Toll-like receptors 1-10 in periodontitis. Oral Microbiology and Immunology. 2008;23(5):425-431. DOI: 10.1111/j.1399-302X.2008.00448.x

[46] Narayan I, Gowda TM, Mehta DS, Kumar BT. Estimation of Toll-like receptor 9 in gingival tissues of patients with chronic periodontitis with or without hyperlipidemia and its association with the presence of *Porphyromonas gingivalis*. Journal of Indian Society of Periodontology. 2018; 22(4): 298-303. DOI: 10.4103/jisp.jisp_124_18

[47] Mori Y, Yoshimura A, Ukai T, Lien E, Espevik T, Hara Y. Immunohistochemical localization of Toll-like receptors 2 and 4 in gingival tissue from patients with periodontitis. Oral Microbiology and Immunology. 2003;18(1):54-58. DOI: 10.1034/j.1399-302x.2003.180109.x

[48] Becerik S, Ozsan N, Gürkan A, Oztürk VO, Atilla G, Emingil G. Toll like receptor 4 and membrane-bound CD14 expressions in gingivitis, periodontitis and CsA-induced gingival overgrowth. Archives of Oral Biology. 2011;56(5):456-465. DOI: 10.1016/j.archoralbio.2010.11.008

[49] Promsudthi A, Poomsawat S, Limsricharoen W. The role of Toll-like receptor 2 and 4 in gingival tissues of chronic periodontitis subjects with type 2 diabetes. Journal of Periodontal Research. 2014;49(3):346-54. DOI: 10.1111/jre.12112

[50] Wilensky A, Segev H, Mizraji G, Shaul Y, Capucha T, Shacham M, Hovav AH. Dendritic cells and their role in periodontal disease. Oral Diseases. 2014; 20(2):119-126. DOI: 10.1111/odi.12122

[51] Machado LR, Ottolini B. An evolutionary history of defensins: a role for copy number variation in maximizing host innate and adaptive immune responses. Frontiers in Immunology. 2015; DOI:10.3389/fimmu.2015.00115

[52] Liu J, Chen J, Du X, Hu L, Chen L. The expression of hBDs in the gingival tissue and keratinocytes from healthy subjects and periodontitis patients. Archives of Oral Biology. 2014;59:193-198. DOI:10.1016/j.archoralbio.2013.11.007

[53] Hazlett L, Wu M. Defensins in innate immunity. Cell Tissue Research. 2011;343:175-188. DOI:10.1007/s00441-010-1022-4

[54] Sallusto F, Lanzavecchia A. Heterogeneity of CD4+ memory T cells: functional modules for tailored immunity. European Journal of Immunology. 2009;39(8):2076-2082. DOI: 10.1002/eji.200939722

[55] Patente TA, Pinho MP, Oliveira AA, Evangelista GCM, Bergami-Santos PC, Barbuto JAM. Human Dendritic Cells: Their Heterogeneity and Clinical Application Potential in Cancer Immunotherapy. Frontiers in Immunology. 2019; DOI:10.3389/fimmu.2018.03176

[56] Walsh LJ, Seymour G J, Savage NW. Oral mucosal Langerhans cells express DR and DQ antigens. Journal of Dental Research. 1986;65(3):390-393. DOI: 10.1177/00220345860650030301

[57] Dereka XE, Tosios KI, Chrysomali E, Angelopoulou E. Factor XIIIa+ dendritic cells and S-100 protein+ Langerhans' cells in adult periodontitis. Journal of Periodontal Research. 2004;39(6):447-452. DOI: 10.1111/j.1600-0765.2004.00764.x

[58] Moughal NA, Adonogianaki E, Kinane DF. Langerhans cell dynamics in human gingiva during experimentally induced inflammation. Journal de Biology Buccale. 1992;20(3):163-167.

[59] Cury PR, Carmo JP, Horewicz VV, Santos JN, Barbuto JA. Altered phenotype and function of dendritic cells in individuals with chronic periodontitis. Archives of Oral Biology. 2013;58(9):1208-1216. DOI: 10.1016/j.archoralbio.2013.03.013

[60] Allam JP, Peng WM, Appel T, Wenghoefer M, Niederhagen B, Bieber T, Bergé S, Novak N. Toll-like receptor 4 ligation enforces tolerogenic properties of oral mucosal Langerhans cells. The Journal of Allergy and Clinical Immunology. 2008;121(2):368-374.e1. DOI: 10.1016/j.jaci.2007.09.045

[61] Séguier S, Godeau G, Leborgne M, Pivert G, Brousse N. Quantitative morphological analysis of Langerhans cells in healthy and diseased human gingiva. Archives of Oral Biology. 2000;45(12):1073-1081. DOI: 10.1016/s0003-9969(00)00069-8

[62] Stelin S, Ramakrishan H, Talwar A, Arun KV, Kumar TSS. Immunohistological analysis of CD1a langerhans cells and CD57 natural killer cells in healthy and diseased human gingival tissue: A comparative study. Journal of Indian Society of Periodontology. 2009;13(3):150-154. DOI: 10.4103/0972-124X.60228

[63] Saglie FR, Pertuiset JH, Smith CT, Nestor MG, Carranza FA Jr, Newman MG, Rezende MT, Nisengard R. The presence of bacteria in the oral epithelium in periodontal disease. III. Correlation with Langerhans cells. Journal of Periodontology. 1987;58(6):417-422. DOI: 10.1902/jop.1987.58.6.417

[64] Gemmell E, Carter CL, Hart DNJ, Drysdale KE, Seymour GJ. Antigen-presenting cells in human periodontal disease tissues. Oral Microbiology Immunology. 2002;17(6):388-393. DOI: 10.1034/j.1399-302x.2002.170609.x

[65] Zavala WD, Cavicchia JC. Deterioration of the Langerhans cell network of the human gingival epithelium with aging. Archives of Oral Biology. 2006;51(12):1150-1155. DOI: 10.1016/j.archoralbio.2006.06.008

[66] Galdiero M, de l'Ero GC, Marcatili A. Cytokine and adhesion molecule expression in human monocytes and endothelial cells stimulated with bacterial heat shock proteins. Infection and Immunity. 1997;65:699-707. DOI: 10.1128/iai.65.2.699-707.1997

[67] Trevani AS, Chorny A, Salamone G, Vermeulen M, Gamberale R, Schettini J, Raiden S, Geffner J. Bacterial DNA activates human neutrophils by a CpG-independent pathway. European Journal of Immunology. 2003;33:3164-174. DOI: 10.1002/eji.200324334

[68] Tsukamoto Y, Usui M, Yamamoto G, Takagi Y, Tachikawa T, Yamamoto M, Nakamura M. Role of the junctional epithelium in periodontal innate defense and homeostasis. Journal of Periodontal Research. 2012;47(6):750-757. DOI: 10.1111/j.1600-0765.2012.01490.x

[69] Zenobia C, Luo XLL, Hashim A, Abe T, Jin L, Chang Y, Jin ZC, Sun JX, Hajishengallis G, Curtis MA, Darveau RP. Commensal bacteria-dependent select expression of CXCL2 contributes to periodontal tissue homeostasis. Cell Microbiology. 2013;15(8):1419-1426. DOI: 10.1111/cmi.12127

[70] Chang AM, Liu Q, Hajjar AM, Greer A, McLean JS, Darveau RP. Toll-like receptor-2 and -4 responses regulate neutrophil infiltration into the junctional epithelium and significantly contribute to the composition of the oral microbiota.Journal of Periodontology.2019;90(10):1202-1212. DOI:10.1002/JPER.18-0719

[71] Hartmann G, Krieg AM. CpG DNA and LPS induce distinct patterns of

activation in human monocytes. Gene Therapy.1999;6:893-903. DOI: 10.1038/sj.gt.3300880

[72] Jiang Y, Mehta CK, Hsu TY, Alsulaimani FF. Bacteria induce osteoclastogenesis via an osteoblast-independent pathway. Infection and Immunity. 2002;70:3143-148. DOI: 10.1128/IAI.70.6.3143-3148.2002

[73] Gallois A, Lachuer J, Yvert G, Wierinckx A, Brunet F, Rabourdin-Combe C, Delprat C, Jurdic P, Mazzorana M. Genome-wide expression analyses establish dendritic cells as a new osteoclast precursor able to generate bone-resorbing cells more efficiently than monocytes. Journal of Bone and Mineral Research. 2010;25(3):661-672. DOI: 10.1359/jbmr.090829

[74] Van Dyke TE. The management of inflammation in periodontal disease.Journal of Periodontology. 2008; 79:1601-1608. DOI: 10.1902/jop.2008.080173

[75] Pascu EI, Pisoschi CG, Andrei AM, Munteanu MC, Rauten AM, Scrieciu M, Taisescu O, Surpățeanu M, Baniță IM. Heterogeneity of collagen secreting cells in gingival fibrosis--an immunohistochemical assessment and a review of the literature. Romanian Journal of Morphology and Embryology. 2015;56(1):49-61.

[76] Hatakeyama J, Tamai R, Sugiyama A, Akashi S, Sugawara S, Takada H. Contrasting responses of human gingival and periodontal ligament fibroblasts to bacterial cell-surface components through the CD14/Toll-like receptor system. Oral Microbiology Immunology. 2003;18(1):14-23. DOI:10.1034/j.1399-302X.2003.180103.x

[77] Franchi L, Park JH, Shaw MH, Marina-Garcia N, Chen G, Kim YG, Núñez G. Intracellular NOD-like receptors in innate immunity, infection and disease. Cell Microbiology. 2008;10(1):1-8. DOI: 10.1111/j.1462-5822.2007.01059.x

[78] Månsson Kvarnhammar A, Tengroth L, Adner M, Cardell LO. Innate immune receptors in human airway smooth muscle cells: activation by TLR1/2, TLR3, TLR4, TLR7 and NOD1 agonists. PLoS One. 2013;8(7):e68701. DOI: 10.1371/journal.pone.0068701

[79] Wilmanski JM, Petnicki-Ocwieja T, Kobayashi KS. NLR proteins: integral members of innate immunity and mediators of inflammatory diseases. Journal of Leukocyte Biology. 2008; 83:13-30. DOI:10.1189/jlb.0607402

[80] Qiu HN, Wong CK, Chu IMT, Hu S, Lam CWK. Muramyl dipeptide mediated activation of human bronchial epithelial cells interacting with basophils: a novel mechanism of airway inflammation. Clinical and Experimental Immunology. 2013;172(1):81-94. DOI: 10.1111/cei.12031

[81] Leissinger M, Kulkarni R, Zemans RL, Downey GP, Jeyaseelan S. Investigating the role of nucleotide-binding oligomerization domain-like receptors in bacterial lung infection. American Journal of Respiratory and Critical Care Medicine. 2014;189(12):1461-1468. DOI: 10.1164/rccm.201311-2103PP

[82] Inohara C, McDonald C, Nuñez G. NOD-LRR proteins: role in host-microbial interactions and inflammatory disease. Annual Review of Biochemistry. 2005;74:355-383. DOI: 10.1146/annurev.biochem.74.082803.133347

[83] Fritz JH, Ferrero RL, Philpott DJ, Girardin SE. Nod-like proteins in immunity, inflammation and disease. Nature Immunology. 2006;7(12):1250-1257. DOI: 10.1038/ni1412

[84] Uehara A, Takada H. Synergism between TLRs and NOD1/2 in oral epithelial cells. Journal of Dental Research. 2008;87:682-686. DOI: 10.1177/154405910808700709

[85] Strober W, Murray P, Kitani A, Watanabe T. Signaling pathways and molecular interactions of NOD1 and NOD2. Nature Reviews Immunology. 2006;6:9-20. DOI:10.1038/nri1747

[86] Eldridge MJ, Shenoy AR. Antimicrobial inflammasomes: unified signaling against diverse bacterial pathogens. Current Opinion in Microbiology. 2015;23:32-41. DOI: 10.1016/j.mib.2014.10.008

[87] Fink SL, Cookson BT. Apoptosis, Pyroptosis, and Necrosis: Mechanistic Description of Dead and Dying Eukaryotic Cells. Infection and Immunity. 2005;73(4):1907-1916. DOI: 10.1128/IAI.73.4.1907-1916.2005

[88] Xue F, Shu R, Xie Y. The expression of NLRP3, NLRP1 and AIM2 in the gingival tissue of periodontitis patients: RT-PCR study and immunohistochemistry. Archives of Oral Biology. 2015;60(6):948-958. DOI: 10.1016/j.archoralbio.2015.03.005

[89] Franchi L, Eigenbrod T, Muñoz-Planillo R, Nuñez G. The inflammasome: a caspase-1-activation platform that regulates immune responses and disease pathogenesis. Nature Immunology. 2009;10:241-247. DOI:10.1038/ni.1703

[90] Pétrilli V, Dostert C, Muruve DA, Tschopp J. The inflammasome: a danger sensing complex triggering innate immunity. Current Opinion in Immunology. 2007;19(6):615-622. DOI: 10.1016/j.coi.2007.09.002

[91] Yilmaz O, Sater AA, Yao L, Koutouzis T, Pettengill M, Ojcius DM. ATP-dependent activation of an inflammasome in primary gingival epithelial cells infected by Porphyromonas gingivalis. Cell Microbiology. 2010;12(2):188-198. DOI: 10.1111/j.1462-5822.2009.01390.x

[92] Dowling JK, O'Neill LAJ. Biochemical regulation of the inflammasome. Critical Reviews in Biochemistry and Molecular Biology. 2012;47(5):424-443. DOI: 10.3109/10409238.2012.694844

[93] Jin T, Perry A, Jiang J, Smith P, Curry JA, Unterholzner L, Jiang Z, Horvath G, Rathinam VA, Johnstone RW, Hornung V, Latz E, Bowie AG, Fitzgerald KA, Xiao TS. Structures of the HIN domain:DNA complexes reveal ligand binding and activation mechanisms of the AIM2 inflammasome and IFI16 receptor. Immunity. 2012;36(4):561-571. DOI: 10.1016/j.immuni.2012.02.014

[94] Bostanci N, Emingil G, Saygan B, Turkoglu O, Atilla G, Curtis MA, Belibasakis GN. Expression and regulation of the NALP3 inflammasome complex in periodontal diseases. Clinical and Experimental Immunology. 2009;157(3):415-422. DOI:10.1111/j.1365-2249.2009.03972.x

[95] Leszczyńska A, Buczko P, Buczko W, Pietruska M.Periodontal pharmacotherapy-an updated review. Adv Med Sci. 2011;56:123-131. doi:10.2478/v10039-011-0044-9

[96] Zuo L, Lucas K, Fortuna CA, Chuang CC, Best TM. Molecular Regulation of Toll-like Receptors in Asthma and COPD. Frontiers in Physiology. 2015; 6: 312. DOI: 10.3389/fphys.2015.00312

[97] Martinsen JT, Gunst JD, Højen JF, Tolstrup M, Søgaard OS. The Use of Toll-Like Receptor Agonists in HIV-1 Cure Strategies. Frontiers in Immunology. 2020; 11: 1112. DOI: 10.3389/fimmu.2020.01112

[98] Meng Z, Chen Y, Lu M. Advances in Targeting the Innate and Adaptive Immune Systems to Cure Chronic Hepatitis B Virus Infection. Frontiers in Immunology. 2020;10:3127. DOI: 10.3389/fimmu.2019.03127

[99] Mackman RL, Mish M, Chin G, Perry JK, Appleby T, Aktoudianakis V, Metobo S, Pyun P, Niu C, Daffis S, Yu H, Zheng J, Villasenor AG, Zablocki J, Chamberlain J, Jin H, Lee G, Suekawa-Pirrone K, Santos R, Delaney WE 4th, Fletcher SP. Discovery of GS-9688 (Selgantolimod) as a Potent and Selective Oral Toll-Like Receptor 8 Agonist for the Treatment of Chronic Hepatitis B. Journal of Medicinal Chemistry. 2020;63(18):10188-10203. DOI: 10.1021/acs.jmedchem. 0c00100

[100] Adams S. Toll-like receptor agonists in cancer therapy. Immunotherapy.2009;1(6):949-964. DOI:10.2217/imt.09.70

[101] Huang L, Xu H, Peng G. TLR-mediated metabolic reprogramming in the tumor microenvironment: potential novel strategies for cancer immunotherapy. Cell Molecular Immunology. 2018;15:428-437. DOI:10.1038/cmi.2018.4

[102] Maheaswari R, Sivasankar K, Subbarayan S. Toll gates: An emerging therapeutic target. Journal of Indian Society of Periodontology. 2014; 18(6): 686-692. DOI: 10.4103/0972-124X.147398

[103] Colotta F, Dower SK, Sims JE, Mantovani A. The type II 'decoy' receptor: a novel regulatory pathway for interleukin 1. Immunology Today. 1994;15(12):562-6. DOI: 10.1016/0167-5699(94)90217-8

[104] Kondo T, Kawai T, Akira S. Dissecting negative regulation of Toll-like receptor signaling. Trends in Immunology. 2012;33(9):449-58. DOI: 10.1016/j.it.2012.05.002

[105] Hajishengallis G. Toll gates to periodontal host modulation and vaccine therapy. Periodontology 2000, 2009;51:181-207. DOI:10.1111-j.1600-0757.2009.00304.x

[106] Banchereau J, Steinman RM. Dendritic cells and the control of immunity. Nature. 1998;392(6673):245-252. DOI: 10.1038/32588

[107] Kanzler H, Barrat FJ, Hessel EM, Coffman RL. Therapeutic targeting of innate immunity with Toll-like receptor agonists and antagonists. Nature Medicine. 2007;13(5):552-9. DOI: 10.1038/nm1589